Updates in Colo-Proctology

Edited by

J.-C. Givel, G.D. Oates, and J.P.S. Thomson

With Contributions by

A. Akovbiantz, P. Buchmann, C.A. Cabre-Martinez, P. Cassell, L. Chapuis, T.C.B. Dehn, A.L. Desai, M.D. Dinneen, A.R. Dixon, M. Dusmet, G.S. Duthie, A. Fiennes, E. Gemsenjaeger, M. Gilg, J.-C. Givel, R.H. Grace, J.D. Hardcastle, M.G. Hartley, R.J. Heald, U. Herzog, S.P.J. Huddy, H.T. Khawaja, W.A. Kmiot, M.-C. Marti, P. Mathey, M.J.C. Matter, R. Mirimanoff, N.J. Mortensen, F. Munier, G.D. Oates, M.C. Parker, J. Pettavel, M. Pinna Pintor, D.A. Rew, E.P. Saraga, P.F. Schofield, J.H. Scholefield, W.P. Schweizer, N.A. Scott, C.T.M. Speakman, U. Stoffel, H. Striffeler, H. Tevaearai, J.P.S. Thomson, H. Thompson, H. Wehrli, and R.G. Wilson

Springer-Verlag
Berlin Heidelberg New York
London Paris Tokyo
Hong Kong Barcelona
Budapest

Jean-Claude Givel, M.D.

Centre Hospitalier, Université Vaudois (CHUV)
Service de Chirurgie
1011 Lausanne, Switzerland

Geoffrey D. Oates, M.D., F.R.C.S.

The General Hospital
Steelhouse Lane
Birmingham, B4 6NH, United Kingdom

James P.S. Thomson

St. Mark's Hospital
City Road
London EC1V 2PS, United Kingdom

with 46 Figures and 60 Tables

ISBN 978-3-540-55327-4 ISBN 978-3-642-51680-1 (eBook)
DOI 10.1007/978-3-642-51680-1

Library of Congress Cataloging-in-Publication Data.
Updates in colo-proctology/edited by J.-C. Givel, G.D. Oates, and J.P.S. Thomson; with contributions by A. Akovbiantz . . . [et al.]. p. cm. Includes bibliographical references and index.

1. Colon (Anatomy) – Diseases – Congresses. 2. Rectum – Diseases – Congresses. 3. Anus – Diseases – Congresses. I. Givel, J.-Cl. (Jean-Cl.), 1946– II. Oates, G.D. (Geoffrey D.) III. Thomson, James P.S. [DNLM: 1. Intestinal Diseases – congresses. WI 400 U66] RC864.U63 1992 616.3'4 – dc20 DNLM/DLC

Typesetting: Best-set typesetter, Ltd., Hong Kong
24/3130 – 5 4 3 2 1 0 – Printed on acid-free paper

Preface

"Updates in Colo-Proctology" covers the proceedings of the Anglo-Swiss Colo-Proctology Meeting held in St Moritz in 1990. The book contains the papers which were presented and discussed there by physicians of the various specialties concerned with the care of patients with diseases of the colon, rectum and anus. The authors, each distinguished in a particular field, have contributed across a wide range of subjects and different disciplines. The topics covered include surgical and investigative techniques, cancer, inflammatory bowel disease and specific infections.

Being familiar with the previous literature, it is clear that little was really new among the themes presented in St Moritz, but few will deny that many of the techniques and methods of treatment described in this book are truly modern. Some contribute an entirely new dimension to the approach to well-known colo-proctological conditions, while others may open up new paths for future research. In addition, in colo-proctology as in other disciplines, advances in treatment almost always bring new problems in the complications which attend them. These are the subject of some of the papers.

Although it would be invidious to pick out individual contributions when there is so much that is new to talk about and so much that is old to be looked at in a new light, we should like to record how much we have enjoyed reading and collating these chapters. We hope that others will share our enthusiasm and pleasure.

Jean-Claude Givel
Geoffrey D. Oates
James P.S. Thomson

Contents

Part I: Technique

Part III: Inflammatory Bowel Diseases

Part IV: Complications

Part V: Miscellaneous

Part VI: Round Tables

Part VII: Posters

List of Contributors

Akovbiantz A. Stadtspital Waid, Tièchestr. 99, 8037 Zürich, Switzerland

Buchmann P. Stadtspital Waid, Tièchestr. 99, 8037 Zürich, Switzerland

Cabre-Martinez C.A. Hospital de Belvitge Princeps d'España, Barcelona, Spain

Cassell P. Spring House, Wexham Street, Stoke Poges SL3 6NK, UK

Chapuis L. CHUV, 1011 Lausanne, Switzerland

Dehn T.C.B. John Radcliffe Hospital, Headington, Oxford OX3 9DU, UK

Desai A.L. Wexham Park Hospital, Slough SL2 4HL, UK

Dinneen M.D. Colchester General Hospital, Turner Road, Colchester, Essex, UK

Dixon A.R. Peterborough District Hospital, Thorpe Road, Peterborough PE3 6DA, UK

Dusmet M. Hôpital de la Chaux-de-Fonds 2400 La Chaux de Fonds, Switzerland

Duthie G.S. Bristol Royal Infirmary, Bristol BS2 8HW, UK

Fiennes A. Rätisches Kantons- und Regionalspital, 7000 Chur, Switzerland

Gemsenjaeger E. Spital Neumünster, 8125 Zollikerberg, Switzerland

Gilg M. Inselspital, 3010 Bern, Switzerland

Givel J.-C. CHUV, 1011 Lausanne, Switzerland

Grace R.H. The Royal Hospital, Wolverhampton WV2 1BT, UK

Hardcastle J.D. University Hospital, Nottingham NG7 2UH, UK

Hartley M.G. Pathology Division, PHLS CAMR, Salisbury, UK

Heald R.J. Basingstoke District Hospital, Basingstoke RG24 9LZ, UK

Herzog U. St. Claraspital, Kleinriehenstr. 30, 4016 Basel, Switzerland

Huddy S.P.J. Basingstoke District Hospital, Basingstoke RG24 9LZ, UK

Khawaja H.T. Royal Sussex Country Hospital, Eastern Road, Brighton BN2 5BE, UK

Kmiot W.A. The Queen Elizabeth Hospital, Edgbaston, Birmingham B15 2TH, UK

Marti M.-C. Hôpital Cantonal Universitaire, 1211 Genève 4, Switzerland

Mathey P. Hôpital Cantonal Universitaire, 1211 Genève 4, Switzerland

Matter M.J.C. Hôpital de Montreux, Service de Chirurgie, 1820 Montreux, Switzerland

Mirimanoff R. CHUV, 1011 Lausanne, Switzerland

Mortensen N.J. John Radcliffe Hospital, Headington, Oxford OX3 9DU, UK

Munier F. Hôpital Ophtalmique, 1004 Lausanne, Switzerland

Oates G.D. The General Hospital, Steelhouse Lane, Birmingham B4 6NH, UK

Parker M.C. St George's Hospital, Blackshaw Road, London SW17 0QT, UK

Pettavel J. CHUV, 1011 Lausanne, Switzerland

Pinna Pintor M. Centro Rieducazione Funzionale, Strada San Vito, Torino, Italy

Rew D.A. 101 Warren Crescent, Shirley Warren, Southampton SO1 6AY, UK

Saraga E.P. Institut Universitaire de Pathologie, 1005 Lausanne, Switzerland

Schofield P.F. Withington Hospital, West Didsbury, Manchester M20 8LR, UK

Scholefield J.H. Flat 3, 344 City Road, London EC1V 2PS, UK

Schweizer W.P. Inselspital, 3010 Bern, Switzerland

Scott N.A. Christie Hospital & Holt Radium Institut, Wilmslow Road, Manchester M20 9BX, UK

Speakman C.T.M. Central Middlesex Hospital, Acton Lane, London NW10 7NS, UK

Stoffel U. Stadtspital Waid, Tièchestr. 99, 8037 Zürich, Switzerland

Striffeler H. Inselspital, 3010 Bern, Switzerland

Tevaearai H. CHUV, 1011 Lausanne, Switzerland

Thomson J.P.S. St. Mark's Hospital, City Road, London EC1V 2PS, UK

Thompson H. The General Hospital, Steelhouse Lane, Birmingham B4 6NH, UK

Wehrli H. Stadtspital Waid, Tièchestr. 99, 8037 Zürich, Switzerland

Wilson R.G. Western General Hospital, Crewe Road, Edinburgh EH4 2XU, UK

Part I: Technique

Endoluminal Sonography as a Preoperative Staging Method for Rectal Cancer

U. Herzog and P. Tondelli

Introduction

The selection of an appropriate surgical procedure for primary rectal cancer depends on the degree of local invasion of the tumour, its mobility, accessibility and size and the presence of involved lymph nodes.

In 1956 Wild and Reid [1] described for the first time the application of an endorectal ultrasound probe as a diagnostic instrument for rectal cancer. But for technical reasons the method did not become attractive until recently when it was used for preoperative staging of rectal cancer [2–6].

This new staging method has aroused major interest because digital examination is highly subjective, its accuracy related to the experience of the investigator. Moreover, tumours in the higher rectum are not within the reach of digital assessment. Another staging method is computed tomography (CT), by which only general assessment of tumour invasion is possible [7]. Accurate prediction of the involvement of different layers of the rectal wall is impossible.

Our experience of digital staging [8] and the unsatisfactory results of CT led to our attempt to achieve a more reliable preoperative assessment of local invasion with endosonography.

Patients and Method

Forty-nine consecutive patients – 28 men, 21 women; mean age 70 (40–93) years – with primary rectal carcinoma were examined preoperatively with an ultrasound scanner type 1846 (Brüel and Kjaer). The endoprobe consists of a rectal tube, a motor unit and a rotating rod, at the end of which a 7.0 MHz (focal length 2–5 cm) 90° transducer is mounted.

All examinations were performed in lithotomy position. The transducer at the tip of the endoprobe – always introduced through a rectoscope – was surrounded with a water-filled balloon for better ultrasonic contact.

With this technique five basic layers of the rectum can clearly be identified – corresponding to the anatomical layers of the rectal wall – as demonstrated by Beynon and Mortensen [9, 10] in in vitro studies. The first hyperechoic layer corresponds to the interface between the water-filled balloon and the mucosal surface; the second hypoechoic layer corresponds to the mucosa and muscularis mucosae; the third hyperechoic layer to the submucosa; the fourth hypoechoic layer to the muscularis propria; and the fifth hyperechoic layer finally represents the interface between the muscularis propria and perirectal fat or peritoneum, if present (Fig. 1). Occasionally the fourth hypoechoic layer may be divided into an inner hypoechoic layer corresponding to the circular muscle coat and an outer hypoechoic layer representing the longitudinal muscle coat; these are separated by a hyperechoic interface [11, 12].

The preoperative ultrasound staging and the postoperative histopathological staging based on the Union International Contre le Cancer (UICC) TNM system [13] were compared. In the TNM system T1 describes a tumour confined to the mucosa or submucosa, T2 a tumour with invasion of the muscularis propria, T3 a tumour with invasion beyond the muscle wall into the perirectal fat or covering peritoneum, and T4 a tumour with infiltration of an adjacent organ.

Results

Of our 49 patients one patient had the tumour removed endoscopically, in five patients the tumour was resected transanally and 43 patients had a laparotomy (24 anterior resections, 17 abdominoperineal excisions and two Hartmann procedures). All 49 resected specimens were examined by the same pathologist.

Using the uT classification described by Feifel [14], in which "u" means ultrasonic and which corresponds well with pathologists' pT classification, we found in the preoperative ultrasonic staging seven cases of uT1 (Fig. 2), nine cases of uT2 (Fig. 3), 33 cases of uT3 and no uT4 carcinoma.

The postoperative pathologic distribution using the above-mentioned TNM staging system revealed: nine cases of pT1, nine cases of pT2, 28 cases of pT3 and three cases of pT4.

Comparing preoperative sonographic assessment with postoperative histopathologic staging we found an accuracy of 82%. In five patients we overestimated the depth of tumour penetration: in three patients the pathologist found pronounced signs of peritumoral inflammation, in one there was a peritumoral abscess, and one patient showed fibrosis after preoperative radiotherapy. In four cases the tumour was understaged: all four patients had a stenotic tumour which could not be passed with the endoprobe, for which reason maximal tumour penetration was probably not assessed (Table 1).

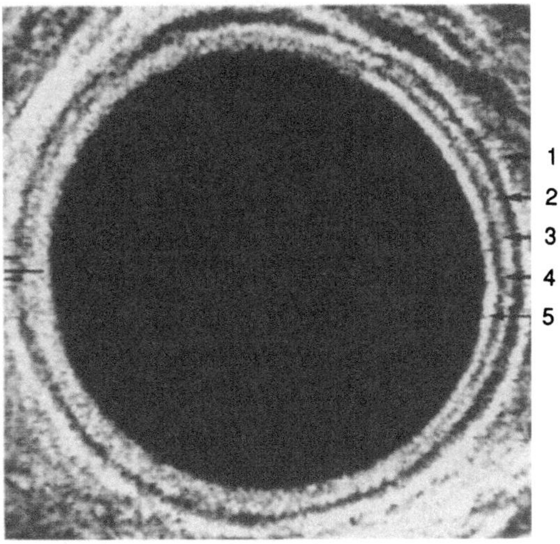

Fig. 1. The five basic layers of the rectum seen through an ultrasound scanner. *1* Interface between water-filled balloon and mucosa, *2* mucosa/muscularis mucosae, *3* submucosa; *4* muscularis propria; *5* interface between muscularis propria and perirectal fat or peritoneum

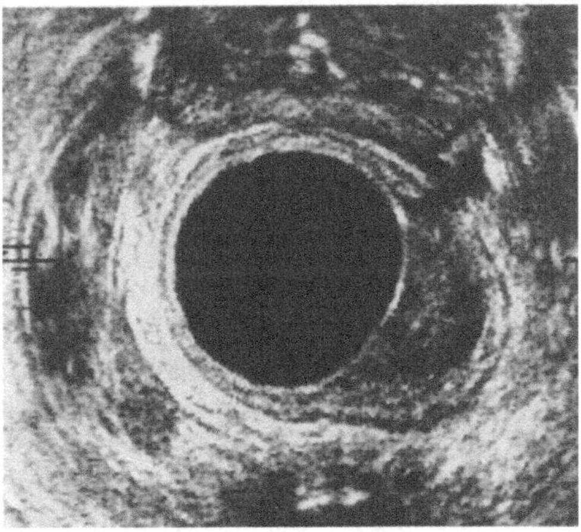

Fig. 2. uT1 carcinoma

For comparison of endoluminal sonography with other preoperative staging methods such as Mason's clinical staging [15] or CT we analysed only those patients within the reach of digital assessment which did not present with a stenotic tumour. We compared results of all these methods with the histopathologic findings. This was possible in 30 patients. In 21 of 30 patients (70%) the clinical staging was correct, in 8 of 30 patients (27%) we overstaged the tumour and in 1 of 30 patients (3%) we underestimated the

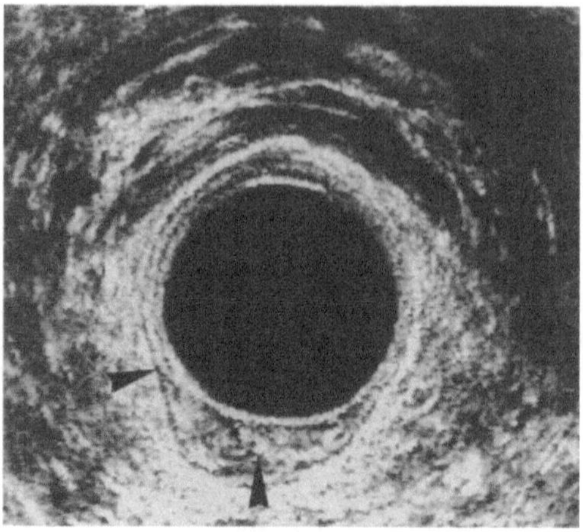

Fig. 3. uT2 carcinoma. *Arrows* show disruption of the submucosa

Table 1. Results with endoluminal sonography (n = 49)

	Ad/pT1	pT2	pT3	pT4
	○			△
uAd/uT1	7			
uT2	2	6	1	
uT3		3	27	3
	□			

Ad, adenoma; □, overstaging; △, understaging; ○, correct staging

true tumour stage. In the same group of patients we had a correct staging with endoluminal sonography in 87% (26/30 patients) and an overstaging in only 4 of 30 patients (13%); there was no understaging. CT was performed in 23 of these 30 patients. A correct preoperative diagnosis was attained in 74%, and in 26% the correct degree of tumour infiltration was not assessed (9% overstaging, 17% understaging) (Table 2).

Discussion

An accuracy of 87% with endoluminal sonography compared with 70% with clinical staging and 74% with CT underlines the value of this new

Table 2. Staging methods compared

	Accuracy (%)	Overstaging (%)	Understaging (%)
CS[a]	70	27	3
CT[b]	74	9	17
EUS[a]	87	13	–

CS, clinical staging; CT, computed tomography; EUS, endoluminal ultrasonography
[a] $n = 30$
[b] $n = 23$

preoperative method in staging rectal cancer. The depth of invasion of a rectal carcinoma in the lower rectum defines the surgical strategy – local excision or resection of the tumour. The treatment of choice for tumours in the middle or upper rectum is anterior resection.

The preoperative digital assessment of rectal carcinoma – first described by Mason [15] – shows a fairly good accuracy of about 60%–75% [3, 8, 16, 17]; but its reliability depends too much on the experience of the examiner. Furthermore it is not reproducible and high tumours in the rectum are out of the reach of the palpating finger. CT scans can demonstrate neither the layered structure of the rectal wall nor small rectal tumours in the lower rectum [18]. In accordance with the UICC TNM system the accuracy of preoperative CT staging is reported to be between 40% and 82% [4, 19–22]. A direct comparison of the reported figures is difficult because clear guidelines for assessment of invasion are not given and the CT technique differs with different scanners.

With endorectal ultrasonography it is possible to visualize the layered structure of the rectal wall. Transducers with a high frequency (7.0–7.5 MHz) permit the visualization of five to seven layers of the rectal wall [12, 23]. The interpretation of the ultrasonic picture of the rectal wall requires a defined relationship between normal histologic structures and the ultrasonic anatomy. In general most authors agree that the five basic layers can be demonstrated clearly: a first hyperechoic layer, a second hypoechoic, a third hyperechoic, a fourth hypoechoic and a fifth hyperechoic layer. But do these five ultrasonic layers correspond to the five histological layers of the rectal wall (mucosa, muscularis mucosae, submucosa, muscularis propria and perirectal fat or peritoneum respectively)? All investigators agree that the fourth hypoechoic layer corresponds to the important muscularis propria. The interpretation of the third hyperechoic layer remains controversial [23–25]. For our study we accepted the interpretation of Beynon et al. [23]. Their anatomically based interpretation is as follows:

1. First hyperechoic layer – interface between water-filled balloon and mucosal surface
2. Second hypoechoic layer – combined image produced by mucosa and muscularis mucosae
3. Third hyperechoic layer – submucosa
4. Fourth hypoechoic layer – muscularis propria
5. Fifth hyperechoic layer – interface between muscularis propria and perirectal fat or peritoneum

In our present study a 7.0 MHz radial scanner was used. The result of the assessment of invasion in 49 patients was satisfactory; overall accuracy was 82%. In all seven patients with an adenoma or pT1 carcinoma the preoperative ultrasonic diagnosis was correct. A differentiation between adenoma and carcinoma was not possible, because the true limiting structure – the muscularis mucosae – could not be visualized. The statement that adenomas are homogeneous and echo-rich while carcinomas are inhomogeneous and echo-poor [26] is an observation which is in general true, but allows no histological diagnosis. As the treatment is the same for both, it is not imperative to distinguish between them.

In the nine patients diagnosed as having uT2 carcinomas, only six were correctly interpreted. Two cases were overstaged, whereby one of these patients showed pronounced peritumoral inflammation, and the other had histologically proven signs of fibrosis after preoperative radiotherapy. Wang [27] presented good results in the assessment of tumours invading the submucosa with a 8.5-MHz linear scanner. The more reliable the distinction of the stages uT1–uT2 the greater the predictive confidence in choosing local excision as treatment. Differentiation between fibrosis and true carcinoma is difficult or even impossible. Similar observations were reported by Mascagni [28] with regard to postoperative fibrosis and tumour recurrence.

In the 33 uT3 carcinomas, three were overstaged, all with pronounced signs of peritumoral inflammation, a condition resembling postoperative fibrosis, with consecutively wrong interpretations of the ultrasound pictures. The three cases which were understaged – as was the case for the patient with understaging in uT2 group – presented a stenotic tumour which could not be passed with the endoprobe, thereby probably not allowing the assessment of maximal tumour penetration.

Our results correspond well to the reported figures in the literature [5, 20, 21, 29]. They confirm the superiority of endoluminal sonography compared with clinical staging or CT. Summarizing the results we may say that the accuracy of clinical staging is about 70%, of CT about 80% and of endoluminal sonography about 90%.

These results illustrate the reliability of a new staging method which will probably facilitate choice of the correct operation (local excision or abdomino-perineal excision) in tumours of the lower rectum.

References

1. Wild JJ, Reid JM (1956) Diagnostic use of ultrasound. Br J Phys Med 19: 248–257
2. Dragsted J, Gammelgaard J (1983) Endoluminal ultrasonic scanning in the evaluation of rectal cancer: a preliminary report of 13 cases. Gastrointest Radiol 8: 367–369
3. Hildebrandt U, Feifel G (1985) Preoperative staging of rectal cancer by intrarectal ultrasound. Dis Colon Rectum 28: 42–46
4. Romano G, De Rosa P, Vallone G, Rotondo A, Grassi R, Santangelo ML (1985) Intrarectal ultrasound and computed tomography in the pre- and postoperative assessment of patients with rectal cancer. Br J Surg 72: S117–119
5. Beynon J, Foy DMA, Roe AM, Temple LN, Mortensen NJMcC (1986) Endoluminal ultrasound in the assessment of local invasion in rectal cancer. Br J Surg 73: 474–477
6. Konishi F, Muto T, Takahashi H, Itoh K, Kanazawa K, Morioka Y (1985) Transrectal ultrasonography for the assessment of invasion of rectal carcinoma. Dis Colon Rectum 18: 889–894
7. Thoeni RF, Moss AA, Schnyder P, Margulis AR (1981) Detection and staging of primary rectal and rectosigmoid cancer by computed tomography. Radiology 141: 135–138
8. Herzog U, Gemsenjäger E, Tondelli P, Schuppisser JP, Gallacchi P (1986) Präoperatives "clinical staging" beim Rektumtumor. Helv Chir Acta 53: 659–661
9. Beynon J, Mortensen NJMcC, Foy DMA, Channer JL, Virjee J, Goddard P (1986) Endorectal sonography: laboratory and clinical experience in Bristol. Int J Colorectal Dis 1: 212–215
10. Beynon J, Foy DMA, Temple LN, Channer JL, Virjee J, Mortensen NJMcC (1986) The endosonic appearances of normal colon and rectum. Dis Colon Rectum 29: 810–813
11. Yamashita Y, Machi J, Shirouzu K, Morotomi T, Isomoto H, Kakegawa T (1986) Evaluation of endorectal ultrasound for the assessment of wall invasion of rectal cancer. Report of a case. Dis Colon Rectum 31: 617–623
12. Konishi F, Ugajin H, Ito K, Kanazawa K (1990) Endorectal ultrasonography with a 7.5 MHz linear array scanner for the assessment of invasion of rectal carcinoma. Int J Colorectal Dis 5: 15–20
13. Spiessl B, Schiebe O, Wagner G (eds) UICC TNM atlas (1984) Springer, Berlin Heidelberg New York
14. Feifel G, Hildebrandt U, Dhom G (1985) Die endorectale Sonographie beim Rectumcarcinom. Chirurg 56: 398–402
15. Mason AY (1976) Rectal cancer: the spectrum of selective surgery. Proc R Soc Med 69: 237–244
16. Nicholls RJ, York Mason A, Morson BC, Dixon AK, Kelsey Fry I (1982) The clinical staging of rectal cancer. Br J Surg 69: 404–409
17. Williams NS, Durdey P, Quirke P, Robinson PJ, Dyson JED, Dixon MF, Bird CC (1985) Pre-operative staging of rectal neoplasm and its impact on clinical management. Br J Surg 72: 868–874
18. Senagore A, Milsom JW, Senagore P, Mazier WP, Scholten DJ, Zydbel P (1988) A comparison between intrarectal ultrasound and CT scanning in staging of experimental rectal tumors. J Surg Res 44: 522–526
19. Rifkin MD, Ehrlich SM, Marks G (1989) Staging of rectal carcinoma: prospective comparison of endorectal US and CT. Radiology 170: 319–322
20. Kramann B, Hildebrandt U (1986) Computed tomography versus endosonography in the staging of rectal carcinoma: a comparative study. Int J Colorectal Dis 1: 216–218
21. Ruf G, Kohlberger E, Rädecke J, Lausen M, Wimmer B, Kirchner R (1989) Präoperatives Staging des Rectumcarcinoms: Endosonographie versus Computertomographie. Langenbecks Arch Chir 374: 164–168

22. Beynon J, Mortensen NJMcC, Foy DMA, Channer JL, Virjee J, Goddard P (1986) Pre-operative assessment of local invasion in rectal cancer: digital examination, endoluminal sonography or computed tomography? Br J Surg 73: 1015–1017
23. Beynon J, Mortensen NJMcC, Rigby HS (1988) Rectal endosonography, a new technique for the preoperative staging of rectal carcinoma. Eur J Surg Oncol 14: 297–309
24. Saitoh N, Okui K, Sarashina H, Suzuki M, Arai T, Nunomura M (1986) Evaluation of echographic diagnosis of rectal cancer using intrarectal ultrasonic examination. Dis Colon Rectum 29: 234–242
25. Hildebrandt U, Feifel G, Schwarz HP, Scherr O (1986) Endorectal ultrasound: instrumentation and clinical aspects. Int J Colorectal Dis 1: 203–207
26. Buess G, Heintz A, Frank K, Strunck H, Kuntz C, Junginger T (1989) Neue endosonographische Untersuchungstechnik zur Verbesserung der Beurteilung kleiner Rectumtumoren. Chirurg 60: 851–855
27. Wang KY, Kimmey MB, Nyberg DA, Mack LA, Haggitt RC, Shuman WP, Franklin DW, Silverstein FE (1987) Colorectal neoplasms: accuracy of US in demonstrating the depth of invasion. Radiology 165: 827–829
28. Mascagni D, Corbellini L, Urciuoli P, Di Matteo G (1989) Endoluminal ultrasound for early detection of local recurrence of rectal cancer. Br J Surg 76: 1176–1180
29. Rifkin MD, Wechsler RJ (1986) A comparison of computed tomography and endorectal ultrasound in staging rectal cancer. Int J Colorectal Dis 1: 219–223

The Stapled Low Colorectal Anastomosis: Our Experience with 342 Patients (1981–1989)

H. Wehrli and A. Akovbiantz

Introduction

The main aims for a surgeon operating for malignancy and other pathological conditions of the rectum and recto-sigmoid region is to preserve continence, to achieve a low recurrence rate and low morbidity and mortality. Mechanical endoluminal stapling devices have been introduced with this in view. The intention of this study was to evaluate the incidence of mortality, morbidity and local recurrence after stapled low colorectal anastomoses performed between 1981 and 1989.

Patients and Methods

Our study reported on 342 patients (57% males, 43% females) with a mean age of 64.1 years; 73.1% of them were suffering from a malignant disease (48% with metastases) and 26.9% presented with diverticular disease or a villous adenoma. The types of operation performed included low anterior resections (38%), resections of the recto-sigmoid colon (25.7%), sigmoid resections (24%), restorative surgery after Hartmann's operation (7.6%), subtotal colectomies (2.9%) and others (1.7%). The mean hospital stay was 21 days. Associated diseases included hypertonia or heart or pulmonary disease (19%); diabetes (5.8%); psychiatric disease (3.4%) and non-colonic cancers (1.2%). The preoperative preparation included a whole gut irrigation (94.4%) and a 24-h antibiotic prophylaxis with tobramycin and metronidazole for elective surgery. The 31-mm cartridge was used in 95% of anastomoses; the double-stapling technique was applied to 8.8% of mostly very low anastomoses [1]. The distance from the anal verge to the anastomosis was 3.5–7 cm in 38%, 7.5–11 cm in 38.9% and 11–15 cm in 23.1% of patients. The patients had their first bowel movement usually after 8.1 days.

Morbidity and Mortality

No patient died during the operation. The perioperative mortality rate (days 1–30) was 2%. These patients died because of cardiac failure or thromboembolism. In the literature the rate varies between 0% and 7% [2–10].

Postoperative complications included wound infection (10.2%), urinary infection (7.9%), haemorrhage (3.5%), pneumonia (2%), bowel obstruction (2%), thromboembolism (1.7%), abscesses (1.5%) and cardiac failure (1.5%).

Intraoperative Complications

The stapled anastomoses are tested intraoperatively with methylene blue injected endorectally. The primary intraoperative leak rate was 8.2%. The leak was either sutured (3.8%) or a new hand-sewn (3.2%) or stapled anastomosis (0.9%) was performed. In one case (0.3%) an abdomino-perineal amputation was unavoidable. A temporary colostomy was performed in 2.3% of patients with primary leaks (the range in the literature is 7%–58% [3, 4, 11, 12]). Most of these leaks were found in anastomoses less than 7 cm above the anal verge (53%) and 87% occurred in cancer patients.

Postoperative Complications

In 3.5% of the patients a postoperative anastomotic leak developed, which was clinically identified. All these patients had their operation for cancer disease and the anastomoses were found less than 7 cm above the anal verge. There was a need for reoperation (drainage) in 0.9%. In only 0.6% of those with colo-cutaneous fistulas did the leak persist until the patient left the hospital (the figures given in the literature differ widely again from 4% to 18% [2–4, 8, 10, 12, 13]). The reoperation rate for complications which are not directly associated with anastomotic leaks was 2.9% (1.7% haemorrhage, 1.2% bowel obstruction).

Follow-Up

In 78.4% of the patients, there was a regular follow-up by their family doctor or a gastro-enterologist [blood tests, rectal examination, endoscopy, carcino-embryonic antigen (CEA), ultrasound, computed tomography (CT-scan). We followed up 92.7% of our patients who underwent operation with the intraluminal stapler for 2–5 years after surgery, with a mean follow-up of 30.4 months. A minimum follow-up period of 2 years was chosen because Morson et al. [5, 14] reported that 80% of local cancer recurrences occur within 2 years after anterior low resection. Complications occurring in the late postoperative period included an anastomotic stenosis rate of 3.8%, which needed endoluminal dilatation for between 4 and 8 months postoperatively. These stenoses are caused by the well-known tendency of stapled anastomoses to shrink (1.6%–14% [2, 3, 7–9, 11, 13]). Persisting colo-cutaneous fistulas were found in 2% of our patients, one third resulting from a primary intraoperative leak. No patient complained of major problems with continence.

At the time of analysis 35% of the cancer patients and only 3.3% of the patients with benign disease were dead, and 84% of them died because of their malignant disease. Of these, 15.8% suffered from a recurrent cancer, whereby the recurrence was within the first 2 years of follow-up in 77.5%. In patients with recurrent cancer 52.5% of the anastomoses were found less than 7 cm from the anal verge. The local recurrence rate after curative and non-curative surgery was the same (16.2% versus 15.4%). According to the results of Glimelius, cited by Malmberg et al. [5], there is no correlation between the local recurrence rate and Dukes' classification. The presence of a postoperative leak or fistula did not influence the recurrence rate (16.7%). Locally recurrent cancer was found after surgery for C2 and D cases in 52.5% of patients, in 5% for C1, in 40% for B2 and in 2.5% for B1 tumors. A total of 27.2% of the patients had metastatic disease; in 76.5% of them, this occurred during the first 2 years, and in 16.4% of them after curative and in 39.6% of them after non-curative resections. The actuarial survival after low rectal stapled anastomosis for cancer in our series is shown in Fig. 1.

Discussion

In experienced hands, the endoluminal stapler has become an important instrument in the preservation of continence in low colorectal disease. The circular stapler has different advantages and disadvantages compared with the hand-sewn technique (see Table 1). There are some technical difficulties including serosal damage during insertion of the instrument (we use Hegar dilatators prior to insertion), instrument failure when firing, incomplete bowel division and anastomotic tears during extraction [3, 9, 13]. Every user of a stapler must be able to cope with these pitfalls and to perform a conventional hand-sewn anastomosis for these reasons. After a world-wide usage for over more than 12 years, one can say that the circular stapler is a

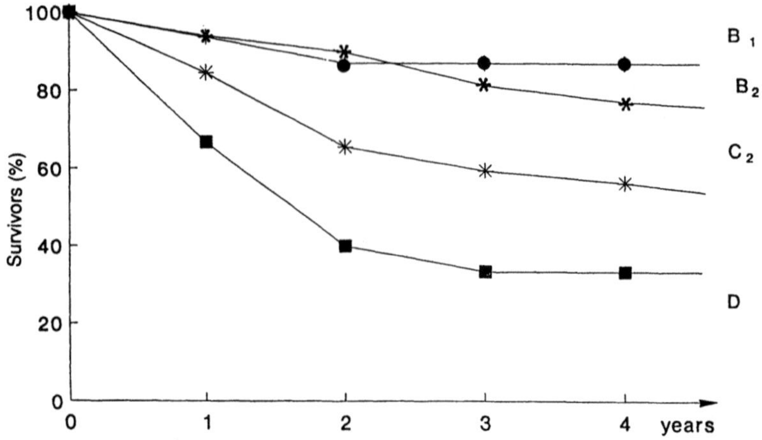

Fig. 1. Actuarial survival after low rectal stapled anastomosis for cancer

Table 1. Advantages and disadvantages of the circular intraluminal stapler (EEA)

Advantages		Disadvantages
Certain	Better vascularisation	Cost
	Lower leakage rate	Rigid anastomosis
	Better tensile strength	Stenosis
		Instrument failure
Uncertain	Time gain	
	Lower anastomosis	
	Shorter hospital stay	

safe instrument which reduces the rate of abdomino-perineal excisions by between 12% and 60% [6, 8]. Controversy still exists over the incidence of local recurrence after stapled anastomoses for rectal cancer [2–6, 8, 10, 11], the difference in leakage rate and the influence of a leak on locally recurrent cancer compared with sutured anastomoses [2, 8]. The high incidence of stenosis, which usually can be dilated, is well known [8, 11, 13]. There is no gain in operating time and hospital stay for patients with stapled anastomoses. We conclude that the stapling device can be used safely whenever technically possible, but never at the cost of cancer cure [5, 9].

References

1. Picciocchi A, d'Ugo DM, Durastante V, Cardillo G (1988) Double stapling technique for low colorectal anastomoses after anterior resection for rectal cancer. Int Surg 73: 19–22
2. Belli L, Beati CA, Frangi M, Aseni P, Rondinara GF (1988) Outcome of patients with rectal cancer treated by stapled anterior resection. Br J Surg 75: 422–424
3. Fazio VW, Jagelman DG, Lavery IC, McGonagle BA (1985) Evaluation of the proximate-ILS^{R} circular stapler. Ann Surg 201: 108–114
4. Gillen P, Peel ALG (1985) Nahtinsuffizienz und Lokalrezidiv nach maschineller Anastomosennaht bei anteriorer Rectumresektion. Coloproctology 4: 220–222
5. Malmberg M, Graffner H, Ling L, Olsson SA (1986) Recurrence and survival after anterior resection of the rectum using the end to end anastomotic stapler. Surg Gynecol Obstet 163: 231–234
6. Odou MW, O'Connell TX (1986) Changes in the treatment of rectal carcinoma and effects on local recurrence. Arch Surg 121: 1114–1116
7. Smith LE (1981) Anastomosis with EEA stapler after anterior colonic resection. Dis Colon Rectum 24: 236–242
8. Waxman BP (1983) Large bowel anastomoses. II. The circular staplers. Br J Surg 70: 64–67
9. Wehrli H, Koch R, Akovbiantz A (1988) Erfahrungen mit 169 maschinellen kolorektalen Anastomosen (1981–1984). Helv Chir Acta 55: 649–654
10. Williams NS, Durdey P, Johnston D (1985) The outcome following sphincter-saving resection and abdomino-perineal resection for low rectal cancer. Br J Surg 72: 595–598
11. Bérard P, Papillon M, Jacquemard R, Labrosse H, Bigay D, Guillemin G (1981) L'anastomose colo-rectale basse à la pince EEA dans la chirurgie du cancer du rectum. A propos de 50 cas. J Chir (Paris) 118: 115–119
12. Everett WG, Friend PJ, Forty J (1986) Comparison of stapling and hand-suture for left-sided large bowel anastomosis. Br J Surg 73: 345–348
13. Testas P, Chollet JM, Lautard M (1987) Les anastomoses mécaniques circulaires colo-rectales par voie trans-anale. A propos d'une série de 51 cas. J Chir (Paris) 124: 241–245
14. Morson BC, Vaughan EG, Bussey HJR (1963) Pelvic recurrence after excision of the rectum for carcinoma. Br Med J 2: 13–18

Is Restorative Proctocolectomy a Viable Alternative in Older Patients?

G.S. Duthie and D.C.C. Bartolo

Introduction

Excellent results are now achieved after restorative proctocolectomy which has become the treatment of choice for younger patients with ulcerative colitis. No results are published for the success of the procedure in older patients who form a smaller but significant group. It may be that the reluctance to perform these procedures in this group of patients relates to the known deterioration of sphincter function with age [1], since continence after this operation depends not only on successful pouch surgery but also on sphincter function, which may be reduced after the surgery. We have undertaken restorative proctocolectomy for ulcerative colitis regardless of age and functionally evaluated the operation in both younger and older groups.

Patients and Methods

Thirty-two patients with ulcerative colitis requiring restorative proctocolectomy were identified (24 male, 8 female; aged 25–73 years) and recruited for study. These patients were sent a questionnaire about pouch function 6 months after the covering ileostomy was closed. Frequency of pouch emptying, both by day and by night were recorded as was any tendency to leak. The ability of the patient to defer emptying of the pouch once this desire was appreciated was also recorded.

The requirement to strain in an attempt to empty, a feeling of improper emptying, urgency of emptying, and the simple awareness of the need to empty was subjectively assessed on a four-point scale:

Event occurring:

Nearly always	(>75% of occasions)
Usually	(50%–75% of occasions)
Occasionally	(25%–50% of occasions)
Almost never	(<25% of occasions)

The use of drugs to reduce emptying frequency was also recorded.

Table 1. Pouch activity

	Young group		Older group	
	Median	Range	Median	Range
Bowel frequency				
Preoperative (per day)	15	3–25	10.5	8–25*
Postoperative (per day)	6	3.5–13	5.5	3–9*
Nocturnal frequency	1	0–4	1	0–2
Deferment interval (h)	2	0.25–12	1.25	0.25–8
Nocturnal leaking (no.)	3		1	

* $p < 0.05$ compared with preoperative values (Wilcoxon)

Results

The patients were divided into two groups, those under 50 years of age (59%; median age 31 years, range 25–50), and those over 50 years (41%; median age 60.5 years, range 51–73). Fifty years was chosen as the dividing age as all other series report on groups under this age, and the aging effect on anal function is more apparent after that age.

Bowel frequency was reduced in the postoperative period (Table 1), but this was to be expected since the majority of these procedures were undertaken as treatment for active colitis. There was no difference in the number of nocturnal emptying events between the groups, nor in the patients' capacity to defer emptying of the pouch. Leakage of pouch contents at night was slightly more prevalent in the younger group, but we must emphasize that this was an occasional occurrence in all cases and not considered by the patients concerned to be socially debilitating. One of our younger patients also suffered minor daytime leakage. Four of the older group and two of the younger group used Imodium® to reduce pouch-emptying frequency.

Pouch function seemed similar in both groups. Table 2 shows all patients had reasonable awareness of the need to empty the pouch, and in only a few instances was this associated with urgency of defaecation. Problems with straining to empty the pouch and feelings of incomplete pouch emptying were similar in both groups, but there was a trend for these to be more prevalent in the older group. This trend did not reach significance.

Discussion

There is a significant reduction in anal function [1] related to age, especially marked in women over 40 years. Laurberg and Swash [2] suggest this

Table 2. Pouch function

	Nearly always (%)	Usually (%)	Occasionally (%)	Almost never (%)
Straining				
Young	7	23	23	47
Older	22	0	11	67
Emptying				
Young	15	60	25	0
Older	44	56	0	0
Urgency				
Young	0	0	46	54
Older	0	0	66	44
Awareness				
Young	85	15	0	0
Older	66	44	0	0

reduction in function relates to the voluntary pressure component, and not to resting pressures. It could be expected that ileal pouch – anal anastomosis would affect resting sphincter function by altering the intrinsic neural pathways of the distal rectum and anal canal. Any reduction of resting pressure would therefore need to be compensated for by voluntary sphincter function. It seems from our work that the degree of compromise of sphincter function after pouch surgery is insufficient to produce a threat to continence, even in the elderly. It seems that the most important factor in function in both groups is the replacement of the diseased rectum with a new more compliant reservoir [3]. The improved storage capacity in the older group presumably negates any deficiencies in sphincter function dependent on age. Our functional assessment shows the older and younger groups are not significantly different with regard to emptying frequency, nocturnal frequency, leakage and the ability to defer pouch emptying. Our older group seems to have slightly more problems with pouch emptying but this is not translated into increased incidence of leakage or nocturnal frequency, although continence has been related to completeness of emptying [4].

It seems from this work that age itself is not a contraindication to restorative proctocolectomy, and we will continue to offer this procedure to our older as well as our younger group of patients.

References

1. McHugh SM, Diamant NE (1987) Effect of age, gender, and parity on anal canal pressures. Contribution of impaired anal sphincter function to fecal incontinence. Dig Dis Sci 32: 726–736
2. Laurberg S, Swash M (1989) Effects of aging on the anorectal sphincters and their innervation. Dis Colon Rectum 32: 737–742
3. Rabau MY, Percy JP, Parks AG (1982) Ileal pelvic reservoir: a correlation between motor patterns and clinical behaviour. Br J Surg 69: 391–395
4. Stryker SJ, Phillips SF, Dozois RR, Kelly KA, Beart RW (1986) Anal and neorectal function after ileal pouch-anal anastomosis. Ann Surg 203: 55–61

Ileo-Anal Reservoir: Our Current Experience

P. Mathey, P. Meyer, J. Robert, P. Morel, D. Mirescu, O. Huber, M.C. Marti and A. Rohner

Introduction

Restorative proctocolectomy with construction of an ileo-anal reservoir has been performed in many patients during the last decade. This technique has proved to be an attractive alternative to the definitive terminal ileostomy in patients suffering from ulcerative colitis or familial polyposis.

Various types of reservoir have been used since Parks' first S-shaped reservoir in 1978 [1]. These include Utsunomiya's J pouch [2], Fonkalsrud's H pouch [3], Nicholls' W pouch [4] and the S-shaped pouch with a short efferent limb [5].

Our experience with ileo-anal reservoirs is based on 40 patients and covers two distinct periods. From 1980 to 1985, we constructed 16 ileo-anal reservoirs: one J- and 15 S-shaped pouches according to Parks' original technique, consisting of a triple-loop S-shaped pouch with a long efferent ileal segment, and an end-to-end anastomosis to the anal canal with a rectal muscular cuff. In time, we changed to S reservoirs with shorter efferent limbs, with the idea of improving spontaneous emptying. From 1986 onwards, we constructed 24 J-shaped reservoirs, making the first important published series of J pouches which reported promising functional results with practically no problems in spontaneous or complete emptying [6, 7].

There were two reasons which led us to abandon the S-shaped pouch despite its otherwise satisfactory function. First, two thirds of our patients (8/11) had difficulty with spontaneous evacuation and reservoir emptying, requiring either the use of a catheter or external massage. Secondly, four patients developed anastomotic or supra-anastomotic stenosis requiring repeated dilatations under general anaesthesia.

We have compared the complications and functional results in patients of both groups. Follow-up ranged from 6 to 114 months with a mean of 54 months since the closure of ileostomy.

Table 1. Complications requiring reoperation

	S Pouch (n = 15)		J Pouch (n = 25)	
	n	%	n	%
Reoperation for early complications	3	20	2	8
Reoperation for late complications	7	47	5	20
Laparotomies	6	40	2	8

Complications

Dehiscences

In the S-pouch group (n = 15), one patient developed an obvious dehiscence with pelvic sepsis which required re-establishment of ileostomy. In the J-pouch group (n = 25), two symptomatic dehiscences occurred: a short, narrow one which rapidly healed with conservative treatment and another one associated with a subphrenic abscess which required drainage under computed tomography (CT) control, but no operation. One asymptomatic anastomotic dehiscence was found by routine radiology in each group, both of which healed spontaneously (Table 1).

Strictures

These were the commonest complications in the S-pouch group. Four patients (27%) developed anastomotic (n = 1) or supra-anastomotic (n = 3) strictures which required repeated dilatation. Strictures occurred in two patients in the J-pouch group.

Postoperative Haemorrhage

One patient in each group required reoperation for haemorrhage occurring the day after performing the reservoir operation.

Small-bowel Obstruction

Three patients with S-pouches developed small-bowel obstruction at 10 days, 1 month and 1 year respectively after closure of their ileostomy and required laparotomy. No obstruction occurred in the J-pouch group.

Other Complications

Three young female patients developed other unusual complications which required reintervention. One case of peritonitis due to perforation of an S pouch more than 3 years after ileostomy closure was treated by suture of the perforation and a new defunctioning ileostomy; the mechanism of perforation was unclear and might have followed an episode of pouchitis in a patient who used a catheter to empty her reservoir. Another patient developed a tumour-like inflammation, 10 cm in diameter, within a J pouch, which required laparotomy, "pouchotomy", and excision. A third patient required reoperation, by a perineal approach, for mucosal prolapse from a J pouch.

Pouchitis

Four patients with S pouches (27%) and four with J pouches (17%) experienced episodes of pouchitis. The incidence of pouchitis will possibly increase with time within the J pouch group.

Failures

A terminal ileostomy had to be reconstructed in two cases (5%), one for perforation of a reservoir and the other for persistent pelvic sepsis due to anastomotic dehiscence.

Functional Results

Reservoir function was assessed in 28 patients: two patients with S pouches were lost to follow-up and two others had ileostomy re-establishment. Eight patients with J pouches were excluded because follow-up after ileostomy closure was less than 12 months. Mean duration of follow-up was 84 months (69–114 months) for the S-pouch group and 32 months (14–75 months) for the J-pouch group (Table 2).

Bowel Movements

Bowel movements (BM) averaged between five and six per 24 h and were slightly more frequent in the J-pouch group, the difference not being significant. One patient in each group had eight to ten BMs per 24 h. Sixteen patients had no nocturnal BM while one in each group had two or three nocturnal BMs.

Table 2. Functional results: emptying

	S Pouch (n = 11)		J Pouch (n = 17)	
	n	%	n	%
Catheter	2	18		0
External massage	6	55		0
Antidiarrhoeal agent	3	27	6	35
Urgency		0		0

Continence

No patient experienced major day-time or night-time incontinence. In the S-pouch group, three patients (27%) had mucous and/or minimal faecal soiling and had to wear pads, either occasionally (n = 1) or regularly (n = 2). In the J-pouch group, 10 patients (57%) had soiling which was usually minimal since only five had to wear pads (regularly two, occasionally three).

Finally, two thirds of the patients in each group never had to wear pads.

Antidiarrhoeal Medication

Three patients with S pouches (27%) and six with J pouches (35%) had to take antidiarrhoeal agents either occasionally or regularly.

Emptying

No patient with a J pouch had any reservoir-emptying problems (Table 1). On the other hand, two thirds of patients with S pouches had difficulties in achieving spontaneous and complete reservoir evacuation: two patients used a catheter and six external massage.

All patients but one were satisfied with their operation and said they would go through it again to avoid a definitive ileostomy.

Conclusion

Early and late complications were lower in the second period (Table 2). Reoperations decreased from 60% in the S-pouch group to 24% in the J-pouch group and the rate of laparotomies for complications fell from 40% to 8%. Such favourable results have been reported in other studies and have probably more to do with increased experience than with the development of new reservoirs [8, 9]. Stenosis of the efferent limb was the most frequent complication in the S-pouch group.

Functional results were slightly better in the S-pouch group. However, most S pouches were performed for familial polyposis (8/11) where results are known to be better [9, 10]. Nearly all J pouches were performed in patients suffering from ulcerative colitis (15/17) and so comparisons are difficult.

Finally, we would like to emphasize, along with several other authors, the drawbacks of performing ileo-anal reservoirs with long efferent limbs. This procedure confers no advantage and may result in poor reservoir function [8, 11, 12].

References

1. Parks AG, Nicholls RJ (1978) Proctocolectomy without ileostomy for ulcerative colitis. Br Med J 2: 85–88
2. Utsunomiya J, Iwama R, Imajo M, Matsuo S, Sawai S, Yaegashi K, Hirayama R (1980) Total colectomy, mucosal proctectomy, and ileoanal anastomosis. Dis Colon Rectum 23: 459–466
3. Fonkalsrud EW (1980) Total colectomy and endorectal ileal pull through with internal ileal reservoir for ulcerative colitis. Surg Gynecol Obstet 150: 1–8
4. Nicholls RJ, Pezim ME (1985) Restorative proctocolectomy with ileal reservoir for ulcerative colitis and familial adenomatous polyposis: a comparison of three reservoir designs. Br J Surg 72: 470–474
5. Vasilevsky CA, Rothenberger DA, Goldberg SM (1987) The S ileal pouch-anal anastomosis. World J Surg 11: 742–750
6. Metcalf AM, Dozois RR, Kelly KA, Beart RW, Wolff BG (1985) Ileal "J" pouch-anal anastomosis. Clinical outcome. Ann Surg 202: 735–739
7. Cohen Z, McLeod RS, Stern H, Grant D, Nordgren S (1985) The pelvic pouch and ileoanal anastomosis procedure. Surgical technique and initial results. Am J Surg 150: 601–607
8. Keighley MRB, Winslet MC, Flinn R, Kmiot W (1989) Multivariate analysis of factors influencing the results of restorative proctocolectomy. Br J Surg 76: 740–744
9. Williams NS, Dozois RR, Goldberg SM, Rothenberg DA, Utsunomiya J, Nicholls RJ, Cohen Z, Hulten LAG, Moskowitz RL (1986) Restorative proctocolectomy with ileal reservoir. Int J Colorectal Dis (symposium) 1: 2–19
10. Becker JM, Raymond JL (1986) Ileal pouch-anal anastomosis. A single surgeon's experience with 100 consecutive cases. Ann Surg 204: 375–381
11. Cohen Z, McLeod RS (1988) Proctocolectomy and ileoanal anastomosis with J-shaped or S-shaped ileal pouch. World J Surg 12: 164–168
12. Nicholls RJ, Gilbert JM (1990) Surgical correction of the efferent ileal limb disordered defaecation following restorative proctocolectomy with the S ileal reservoir. Br J Surg 77: 152–154

Rectal Resection with Coloanal Anastomosis for Carcinoma of the Rectum

E. GEMSENJAEGER

Introduction

In the management of rectal cancer a coloanal anastomosis may be performed when it is technically difficult or impossible to construct a very low colorectal anastomosis from the abdomen, or when adequate curative resection would require total resection of the rectum, but not removal of the pelvic floor and anus [1–13].

Technical variations govern the approach, which may be abdominotransanal [4, 6, 8–13], abdominotranssphincteric [1, 7] or abdominotranssacral [3, 5]. A sleeved anastomosis is performed when a rectal stump remains, or when an overlapping anastomosis, with the colon placed into a rectal or anal sleeve (Fig. 1), is judged to be a safe procedure [2, 8, 9, 11, 12]; end-to-end anastomosis at the anorectal junction is performed when the level of transection is low (Fig. 1) [4, 6, 10, 12, 13]. A stapling device has been used by some surgeons [6, 7], others prefer a hand-sewn anastomosis at the level of the internal anal sphincter [13–15]. Distal bowel transection is usually performed from the abdomen [2, 4, 6, 9–13]; a combined abdominal transanal approach [8], or transection as a preliminary step through the anus [16] with the tumour margin under direct vision or from a posterior, translevator approach [17] has also been used.

In this paper, we report on abdominotranssphincteric and abdominotransanal total rectal resection with coloanal end-to-end anastomosis (Fig. 1).

Surgical Technique

The abdominotranssphincteric resection was performed according to Mason [1], with a diverting colostomy in all cases. The technique of abdominotransanal resection has been standardized in recent years [23]. The splenic flexure is mobilized; the rectum is then mobilized down to the pelvic floor, cross-clamped and transected at the anorectal junction, or even at the level of the internal anal sphincter. The anal stump is cleaned. With

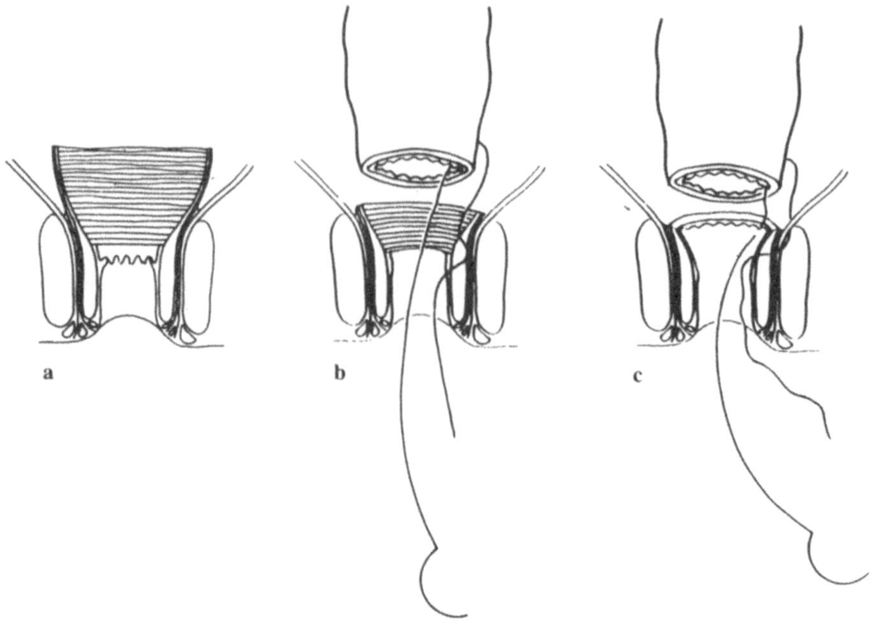

Fig. 1a-c. Coloanal anastomosis with mucosectomy and visceral (**a**, rectal; **b**, anal) sleeve. **c** Coloanal end-to-end anastomosis (somatic muscle sleeve by the pelvic floor muscles)

the patient placed in the lithotomy position the anus is exposed by four traction sutures (Fig. 2) and by a simple anal speculum. All stitches for the anastomosis are first inserted into the anal canal (Fig. 3). They comprise the full thickness of the internal sphincter, the longitudinal muscle, and also a bite of the somatic sphincter funnel (Fig. 1). The colon is then brought to the anus, and the sutures are inserted into the colonic wall, first posteriorly, with the speculum placed in the anal canal (Fig. 4). All sutures are left untied; thereby access and insertion is facilitated. For inserting the anterior stitches the speculum is placed into the colon lumen (Fig. 5). The speculum is then withdrawn and the sutures are tied.

Patients

From 1976 to 1988 total restorative rectal resection for carcinoma with end-to-end coloanal anastomosis was performed in 37 patients. An abdominotranssphincteric resection (n = 13) was performed mostly in the first years of the study; abdominotransanal resection has become the preferred procedure since 1981. The study comprised 28 men and 9 women, aged 37–84 (mean 60) years.

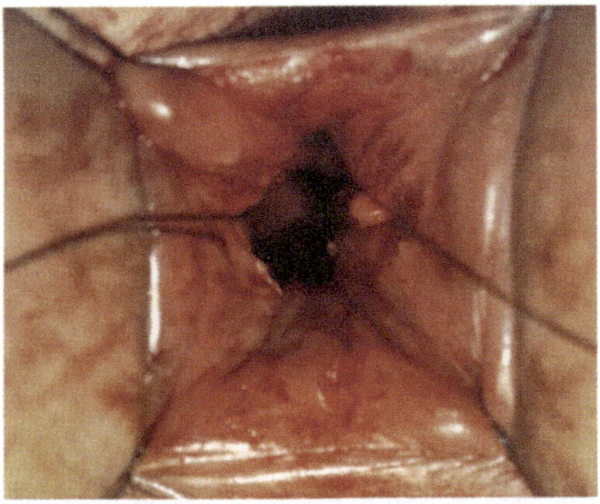
2

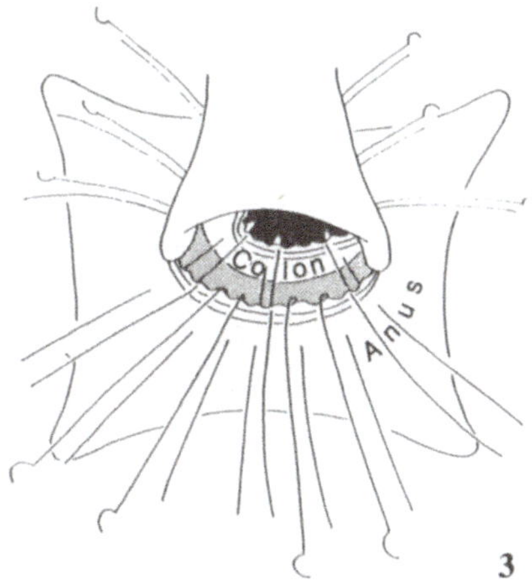

3

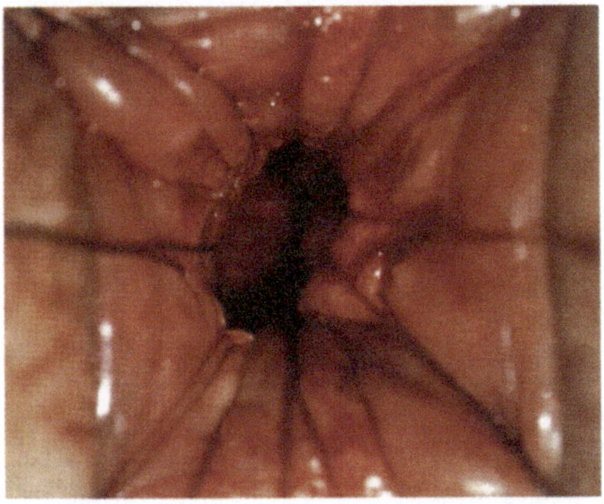
4

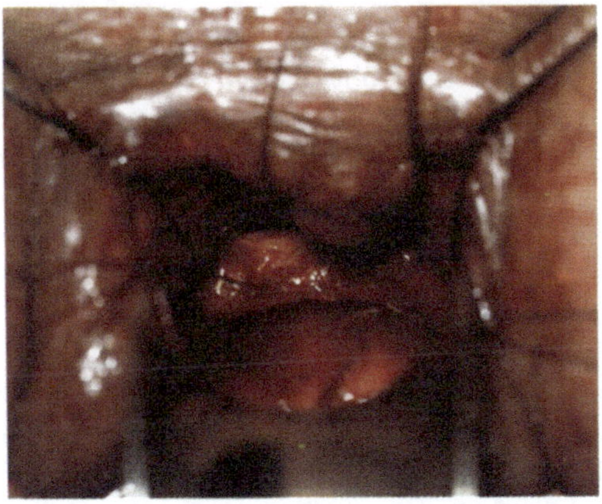
5

Fig. 2. Anus exposed by four traction sutures. Sutures for the anastomosis inserted at 3 and 9 o'clock

Fig. 3. Sutures inserted in the anal canal

Fig. 4. Insertion of sutures into colonic wall; posterior circumference

Fig. 5. Insertion of sutures into colonic wall, anterior circumference

Table 1. Tumour distance from the anal verge[a]

Distance (CM)	No. of patients
5	2
6	15
7	10
8	5
9	3
10	2

[a] Mean ± SD, 6.9 ± 1.3

Table 2. Oncologic results

	No. of patients	Death from disease		Pelvic recurrence	
		n	%	*n*	%
Dukes stage					
A	11	1	9	2	18
B	5	1	20	1	20
C1	7	1	42[a]	2	25
C2	5	4		1	
D	4	4	100[a]	0	0
	32	11		6[b]	19

[a] 0.9–5.0 ($\bar{x}$ = 1.9) years postoperatively
[b] 0.3–2.5 ($\bar{x}$ = 1.3) years postoperatively

The Dukes staging was A 35%, B 16%, C 38%, D (liver metastases) 11%. The mean distance of the tumour from the anal verge was 6.9 (range 5–10) cm (Table 1). The margin of distal clearance on the fresh specimen ranged from 1–5 (mean 2.3) cm.

Results

There was one postoperative death (2.7%). A 70-year-old man died from pelvic sepsis 6 weeks after abdominotranssphincteric resection. Anastomotic leakage and pelvic sepsis occurred in 30% of patients, with clinical significance in 19%; the rate was 38% after abdomino-transsphincteric, and 25% after abdominotransanal resection. Eleven selected patients of the latter group had no colostomy, with pelvic sepsis and secondary colostomy in one case (9%). In no patient was stricture formation observed.

Table 3. Pelvic recurrence

	Number of factors[a] demonstrated by patients			
	0	1	2	3
Patients with pelvic recurrence (n = 6)	0	3	2	1
Patients without pelvic recurrence (n = 26)	6	6	13	1

[a] Possible adverse factors include extent of circumferential growth (≥3 vs <3 quadrants); distance from anal verge (≤6 cm vs >6 cm); and distal margin of clearance (≤2 cm vs >2 cm)

Oncologic Results

One patient was lost to follow-up, one patient died by accident. In two patients operated on for a Dukes C1 tumour early in the series, secondary abdominoperineal excision was indicated because of an unclear distal margin on histology. Thirty-two patients were followed up for 1–9 (mean 3.8) years, or until cancer-related death, which occurred 0.5–5 [1, 9] years postoperatively (Table 2). Six patients (19%) developed a pelvic recurrence, at a mean of 1.3 years postoperatively. All had a secondary abdominoperineal excision. Four of these patients have died. Possible adverse factors (≥ three quadrants involved; ≤6 cm distance from the anal verge; ≤2 cm distal margin) did not appear to influence pelvic recurrence (Table 3).

Functional Results

Only patients with a competent sphincter function were selected for the procedure. One year postoperatively 78% of the eligible patients had a satisfying functional result. A permanent diversion was performed in two patients because of postoperative radiation damage (Table 4).

Discussion

Our results are in agreement with previous reports showing that total rectal resection with coloanal anastomosis is a safe procedure in selected patients [1–12] (Table 5). The operative mortality and morbidity are comparable

Table 4. Functional results[a]

Patients		Result
n	%	
18	64	Normal continence
4	14	Minor defects
3	11	Acceptable, minor leakage, pad
1	4	Major soiling
2	8	Permanent diversion (postoperative radiation therapy)

[a] Group of 28 preoperatively selected patients

Table 5. Rectal resection for carcinoma with coloanal anastomosis

Author	No. of patients	Operative mortality (%)	Pelvic sepsis (%)	Vaginal fistula (%)	Stenosis (%)	Favourable continence (%)	Pelvic recurrence (%)
Bernard [11]	29	0	–	–	44	87	12.5
Drake [9]	19	0	5	–	31	84	6
Enker [6]	41	0	17	–	–	64	–
Hautefeuille [10]	35	0	20	3	0	97	20
Killingback[a]	43	2	–	–	–	50	–
Lazorthes [7]	57	0	9	–	2	80	6
Sweeney [12]	84	2.4	48	2	18	72	18
Wunderlich [8]	24	7.5	20	5	15	80	–
Present series	37	2.7	19	3	0	78	19

[a] Cited by McDermott [4]

to anterior resection or abdomino-perineal excision, but comparisons are difficult because of patient selection and the low number of patients. Pelvic recurrence (with or without disseminated disease) occurred with a variable incidence, depending probably on several factors such as patient selection, follow-up, radiation therapy [5–7], possibly the operative technique and surgeon [18]. In our patients with a Dukes stage C or D tumour, a local (pelvic) recurrence was observed in 19%. Favourable local control in patients with advanced cancer has been demonstrated by others [5–7, 9]. The results reflect the effectiveness of the procedure quite separately from the incidence of early death due to disseminated disease (which in our series occurred later than local recurrence). Local recurrence following radical surgery in Dukes A cancer, which occurred in two (18%) of our patients, is unusual. Our experience may reflect a learning curve with respect to patient selection and technical performance [4]. Achieving a good (≥2 cm) distal margin not only prevents inadequate longitudinal (and lateral) excision [10] but allows for a good distal occlusion of the specimen. Tumour cell spillage from the lumen is one of the hazards inherent in restorative procedures, possibly contributing to a slightly increased recurrence rate reported following restorative operations as compared with abdomino-perineal excision [19]. Technical factors remain important though some statistical results indicate that a small distal margin does not affect local control [19, 20], or survival [21], and that it may even protect from distant spread [22]. Local failure often indicates inadequate primary surgery, whereas distant failure appears to be a sign of unfavourable biological behaviour (as in breast cancer) [21].

After the introduction of a standard transanal anastomotic technique, leaks were observed less frequently [23]. In our experience a single-layer interrupted longitudinal suture technique [24] is ideal for coloanal anastomosis, i.e. at the level of the fixed and thick anal canal wall with the internal anal sphincter. The end-to-end anastomosis comes to lie within a kind of sleeve formed by the somatic muscular funnel. Stricturing of the anastomosis occurred rarely in the series with an end-to-end anastomosis [7, 10]; this was observed more frequently after a visceral sleeve anastomosis [8, 9, 11, 12] (Table 5). In selected cases the distal transsection is performed as a preliminary step from a posterior approach [17]. It permits precise localization of the distal and lateral tumour margins and of the line of resection.

Our functional results with good continence in 78% of patients are comparable with previous reports (Table 5). Preoperative clinical evaluation of the sphincter function (basal and squeeze contraction) was shown to be adequate for the selection of patients with respect to predicting postoperative continence. Postoperative radiation therapy may lead to damage, necessitating permanent diversion [9]. Therefore radiation therapy should be administered preoperatively [5, 7].

Total rectal resection with coloanal end-to-end anastomosis may be offered to patients with a mid-rectal cancer as low as 6 cm from the anal verge, instead of a compromised anterior resection or an abdominoperineal excision. Large and penetrating tumours beginning at 5 cm or below are not suitable for the procedure. At this level the visceral muscle coat becomes fused with the pelvic floor [17]. Small tumours not penetrating rectal wall may be suitable even at 5 cm, as an alternative also to local excision. Distant disease is not a contraindication to total restorative rectal resection.

References

1. Mason AY (1974) Trans-sphincteric surgery of the rectum. Prog Surg 13: 66–97
2. Parks AG, Percy JP (1982) Resection and sutured colo-anal anastomosis for rectal carcinoma. Br J Surg 69: 301–304
3. Localio SA, Eng K, Coppa GF (1983) Abdominosacral resection for midrectal cancer. Ann Surg 198: 320–324

4. McDermott FT (1983) Carcinoma of the rectum. In: Hughes E, Cuthbertson AM, Killingback MK (eds) Colorectal surgery. Churchill Livingstone, Edinburgh, pp 377–379
5. Marks G, Mohiuddin M, Borenstein BD (1985) Preoperative radiation therapy and sphincter preservation by the combined abdominotranssacral technique for selected rectal cancers. Dis Colon Rectum 28: 565–571
6. Enker WE, Stearns MW, Janov AJ (1985) Peranal coloanal anastomosis following low anterior resection for rectal carcinoma. Dis Colon Rectum 28: 576–581
7. Lazorthes F, Fages P, Chiotasso P, Bugat R (1986) Synchronous abdominotranssphincteric resection of low rectal cancer: new technique for direct colo-anal anastomosis. Br J Surg 73: 573–575
8. Wunderlich M, Karner-Hanusch J, Schiessel R (1986) Results of coloanal anastomosis. A prospective study. Int J Colorectal Dis 1: 157–161
9. Drake DB, Pemberton JH, Beart RW, Dozois RR, Wolff BG (1987) Coloanal anastomosis in the management of benign and malignant rectal disease. Ann Surg 206: 600–605
10. Hautefeuille P, Valleur P, Perniceni T, Martin B, Galian A, Cherqui D, Hoang C (1988) Functional and oncologic results after coloanal anastomosis for low rectal carcinoma. Ann Surg 207: 61–64
11. Bernard D, Morgan S, Tasse D, Wassef R (1989) Preliminary results of coloanal anastomosis. Dis Colon Rectum 32: 580–584
12. Sweeny JL, Ritchie JK, Hawley PR (1989) Resection and sutured peranal anastomosis for carcinoma of the rectum. Dis Colon Rectum 32: 103–106
13. Gemsenjäger E (1984) Zur Operationstechnik der abdomino-transanalen Rektumentfernung. Chirurg 55: 670–676
14. Hawley PR (1983) Peranale Anastomose. In: Reifferscheid M (ed) Rektumkarzinom, Sphinktererhaltende Operationsverfahren: Indikation, Technik und Prognose. Thieme, Stuttgart, pp 72–78
15. Allan A, Keighley MRB (1988) Operative approaches to the distal rectum. In: Decosse JJ, Todd IP (eds) Anorectal surgery. Clin Surg Int 15: 213–238
16. Basso N, Minervini S, Marcelli M (1987) Modified abdominotransanal resection for cancer of the lower third of the rectum. Dis Colon Rectum 30: 641–643
17. Gemsenjäger E (1989) Transverse pelvic floor division for the posterior approach to the rectum and anus. Int J Colorectal Dis 4: 67–72
18. Phillips RKS, Hittinger R, Blesovsky L, Fry JS, Fielding LP (1984) Local recurrence following curative surgery for large bowel cancer: II. The rectum and rectosigmoid. 12–16
19. Phillips RKS, Hittinger R, Blesovsky L, Fry JS, Fielding LP (1984) Local reccurence following curative surgery for large bowel cancer: II. The rectum and rectosigmodi. Br J Surg 71: 17–20
20. Pollett WG, Nicholls RJ (1983) The relationship between the extent of distal clearance and survival and local recurrence rates after curative anterior resection for carcinoma of the rectum. Ann Surg 198: 159–163
21. Wolmark N, Fisher B (1986) An analysis of survival and treatment failure following abdominoperineal and sphincter-saving resection in Dukes' B and C rectal carcinoma. Ann Surg 204: 480–489
22. Rinnert-Gongora S, Tartter PI (1989) Multivariate analysis of recurrence after anterior resection for colorectal carcinoma. Am J Surg 157: 573–576
23. Gemsenjaeger E (1988) Anastomosierungstechnik am Anus. Helv Chir Acta 55: 663–666
24. McGinn FP, Gartell PC, Clifford PC, Brunton FJ (1985) Staples or sutures for low colorectal anastomoses: a prospective randomized trial. Br J Surg 72: 603–605

A Prototype Anal Continence Plug

N.J. Mortensen, S. Humphreys, and A. Ballan

Introduction

There is increasing dissatisfaction with the longer term results of anal incontinence surgery [1–7]. In some cases less than 50% of patients retain complete continence 2 or 3 years after surgery. Minor imperfections of continence persist after a range of colorectal procedures. Conservative management with a low residue diet and antidiarrhoeal medication such as codeine phosphate and Imodium® has limited value in patients with gross incontinence [4]. We have therefore designed a prototype anal continence plug. Using a similar principle and similar materials to those employed for the Conseal colostomy plug, the plug, shaped like a champagne cork, is made of polyvinyl alcohol sponge and the stem coated in a lubricated cover which dissolves on placement in the anal canal (Fig. 1). The appliance then gently expands to size to fill the anal canal. It is disposable so that when the subject appreciates an evacuatory desire the plug can simply be expelled by raised intrabdominal pressure and the defaecatory reflex.

Patients and Methods

Nine patients (seven women, two men) with major anorectal incontinence, median age 45 years (range 18–82) agreed to enter the study. Their ages and the aetiology of their incontinence is shown in Table 1. A trained nurse counselled each patient in the insertion and use of the plugs, and they each kept a diary recording ease of insertion, duration of placement and reason for plug expulsion. Two types of plug were trialled, with and without adhesive on the flange. All subjects discontinued antidiarrhoeal medication.

Results

Four patients had an excellent result, with complete continence using 25 plugs for a median 7 h each (range 1.25–24 h). Five other patients had a less

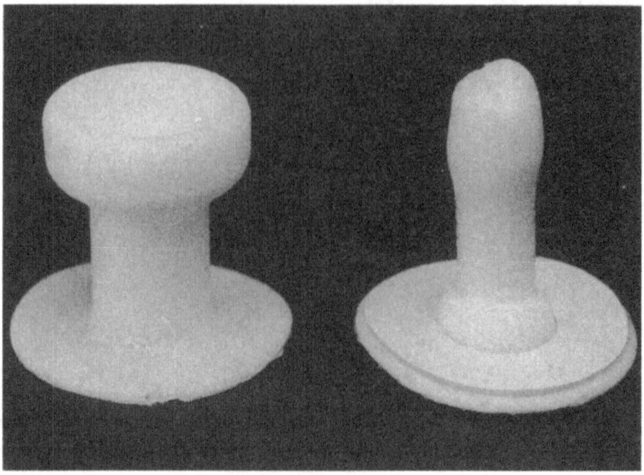

Fig. 1. The prototype anal plug. On the *right* the plug wrapped in water soluble film; on the *left* the expanded plug

favourable experience using 18 plugs for a median 0.4 h (range 0.08–4 h). Reasons given for early plug expulsion were anal canal discomfort (2 patients), easy expulsion (1), diarrhoea (1) and difficulty with plug insertion. Plugs with adhesive were generally retained for longer than those without. Patients with diminished anal canal and rectal sensation tolerated the plugs better than those with normal sensation.

Discussion

Anorectal incontinence is a distressing complaint for the patient and a major management problem for the colorectal surgeon. In the attempt to avoid a colostomy, conservative and operative methods have been advocated. There is no active pharmacological agent with a direct effect on the anal sphincter. The constipating drugs are helpful but not always effective [4]. A diet low in residue will result in less gassy, and less bulky stools which can certainly help the patient with minor incontinence. Although initial results of perineal surgery, whether as a postanal repair or an anterior repair are encouraging, there are an increasing number of operative failures with time [1–7]. It was for these reasons that we introduced this anal continence plug. Four of our nine trial patients were delighted with the confidence the plug gave them, and all wanted further supplies of the plug should it become available. The other five patients were much less impressed. One should not have been recruited to the study in the first place, finding the notion of placing some-

Table 1. Anal continence plug trial: clinical details

Patient	Sex	Age	Diagnosis	Time each plug in place (h)	Comment
1	F	82	Prolapse and incontinence	0.5,0.75,1.25,1	Painful and uncomfortable
2	M	19	Spina bifida	24,24,24,8,24	Delighted, preferred adhesive, activities normal
3	M	45	Spinal injury	24,24,24,24,24	Pleased, preferred adhesive, activities normal
4	F	22	Spinal lipoma	4,1,5,5,5	Fell out easily, adhesive made no difference, burning sensation
5	F	64	Idiopathic incontinence	0.4,0.2,0.2,0.2, 0.2	Off codeine phosphate, developed diarrhoea, couldn't retain plug
6	F	50	Incontinence after postanal repair	1.5,1.25,2,1.5,7 3,2,3,2,3.25	Quite pleased, but plugs caused urge to defaecate, once leaked through flange
7	F	50	Incontinence after postanal repair	0.25,3	Stinging in situ, sore anus, colic
8	F	34	Obstetric injury	0.08,0.5	Although agreed to try found plug distasteful, discontinued
9	F	18	Spina bifida	12,8,7,6.5,7.5	Very pleased

Two types of plug were trialled, one with and one without adhesive on the flange thing in the anal canal distasteful. This is not however a very common reaction. The other four patients were asked to stop their constipating medication during the study which was in retrospect a mistake. Normal rectal and anal canal sensation may result in rectal contractions expelling the plug from the anal canal, perhaps due to its local stimulatory effect. Nevertheless, even if only half of the population of patients with anorectal incontinence were helped with such a device the result would be encouraging.

Development of this plug, used in combination with antidiarrhoeal medication may have a useful place in the management of anorectal incontinence.

References

1. Browning GGP, Parks AG (1983) Postanal repair for neuropathic faecal incontinence: correlation of clinical result and anal canal pressures. Br J Surg 70: 101–104
2. Henry MM, Simson JNL (1985) Results of postanal repair: a retrospective study. Br J Surg 72 [Suppl]: 17–19
3. Keighley MRB (1984) Postanal repair for faecal incontinence. J R Soc Med 77: 285–288
4. Miller R, Bartolo DDC, Locke-Edmunds JC, Mortensen NJMcC (1988) Prospective study of conservative and operative treatment for faecal incontinence. Br J Surg 75: 101–105
5. Womack NR, Morrison JFB, Williams NS (1988) Prospective study of the effects of postanal repair in neurogenic faecal incontinence. Br J Surg 75: 48–52
6. Keighley MRB, Fielding JWL (1983) Management of faecal incontinence and results of surgical treatment. Br J Surg 70: 463–468
7. Laurberg S, Swash M, Henry MM (1990) Effects of post anal repair on progress of neurogenic damage to the pelvic floor. Br J Surg 77: 519–522

Gastro-Intestinal Anastomosis with Continuous Single-Layer Suture Versus Two Layers: A Prospective Randomized Study

W.P. Schweizer, H. Striffeler, P. Gertsch, and L.H. Blumgart

Introduction

Ever since surgeons have been operating within the abdominal cavity, the wide variety of techniques for gastro-intestinal anastomosis have been the object of ongoing discussion. The ideal anastomotic technique must be atraumatic, waterproof, simple, easily learned and rapidly performed. Regardless of the method or suture material, the basis of anastomotic healing is an adequate blood supply, gentle handling of the tissues, tension-free approximation of cut ends of the bowel, good preoperative mechanical bowel preparation and antibiotic prophylaxis. As early as 1887 Halsted [1] reported good results in animal experiments with a single-layer intestinal anastomosis. Allen in 1979 [2] and Bailey in 1981 [3] and 1984 [4] reported satisfactory results with a continuous single-layer polypropylene colorectal anastomosis. These results, a preliminary experience with continuous single-layer anastomosis with a coated woven thread and the introduction of the atraumatic, resorbable, monofil 4/0 polydioxanon (PDS) suture (Ethicon, Edinburgh, UK) encouraged us to evaluate the continuous single-layer suture technique versus the previously routinely used double-layer suture technique in a prospective randomized study. Prior to the start of this study, the new technique was used in an initial learning phase of 3 months.

Patients and Methods

After an introductory learning phase of 3 months, we instituted a prospective randomized trial including all "reversible" small-bowel and right and left colon anastomoses. Emergencies and elective procedures were included. During a 15-month period, 103 anastomoses (17 emergencies, 86 electives) were performed. Patient groups were similar for age, sex and underlying disease. Thirteen patients had an ileus, and in 32 patients a complete mechanical bowel preparation was not possible. All patients received "single shot" antibiotic prophylaxis with a cephalosporin, and for the colon an antianaerobic agent was added. In 26 patients the antibiotic cover was prolonged for various reasons. Fifty-one continuous single-layer anastomoses and 52 double-layer anastomoses were performed. These were distributed amongst 21 small-bowel anastomoses (14 single-layer continuous and 7 double-layer), 44 Roux-en-Y end-to-side anastomoses (18 single-layer continuous and 26 double-layer), six ileotransverse anastomoses after ileocaecal or right colon resection (2 single-layer continuous and 4 double-layer) and 32 colon anastomoses (17 single-layer continuous and 15 double-layer). Ten anastomoses were performed by residents, 69 by senior registrars and 24 by consultants. The time for the anastomosis was taken from the first stitch at the mesenteric border to the last knot of the anastomosis. The leakage rate was assessed by clinical judgement.

Techniques

Single-Layer Anastomosis

After loose approximation of the cut ends of the bowel and using a double-ended 4/0 PDS suture, the mesenteric stitch is placed with two knots. The two ends of the suture are kept with the needle and must be the same length. The continuous suture takes approximately 3-mm bites in the *seromuscular* layer starting on the anterior wall towards the antimesenteric side. The bowel is turned around and the same procedure used for the posterior aspect. The ends are then tied with seven knots on the antimesenteric side. In exceptional cases the continuous single-layer suture may be performed by the technique of posterior followed by anterior wall suturing. This requires care in taking adequate bites on either side of the wall.

Double-Layer Anastomosis

Firstly a *mucosal/submucosal* continuous layer suture starting on the mesenteric side is performed but using an atraumatic resorbable 4/0 suture (Vicryl). At the end of the internal row, an external *seromuscular* interrupted suture is performed using the same material.

On completing each anastomosis the surgeons recorded the technique used and the achieved result as "perfect" or "less than satisfactory". Immediately postoperatively the surgeons also filled in the protocol, including the time needed for the anastomosis.

Table 1. Mean time needed to perform single- and double-layer sutures

	Single (min)	Double (min)
Small bowel	11	23
Roux-en-Y	12	24
Ileocaecal	19	23
Colon	15.5	23

Table 2. Comparison of technique and result for single- and double-layer sutures

	Perfect	Less satisfactory
Single layer	41	7
Double layer	16	36

Results

No clinical leakage occurred throughout the 103 anastomoses. The mean time needed to perform a continuous anastomosis was 11 min for the small bowel versus 23 min for the double layer; 12 min for a Roux-en-Y end-to-side continuous anastomosis versus 24 min for the double layer; 19 min for an ileotransverse continuous anastomosis versus 23 min for the double layer; and 15.5 min for a colon continuous anastomosis versus 23 min for the double layer (Table 1).

Surgeons with varying levels of expertise considered the continuous anastomosis superior to the double-layer suture in most cases (Table 2). There were only a few minor infective complications in both groups. There was no 30-day mortality.

Discussion

For many years the safety and simplicity of the single-layer interrupted anastomotic technique has been advocated by experimental [1, 5–7] and clinical studies [8–11]. Nevertheless the most frequently used method all over the world is still the traditional two-layer method of intestinal anastomosis.

Safe gastro-intestinal anastomosis requires careful handling of the bowel wall, a good blood supply and tension-free approximation of the cut ends of the viscera. Regardless of the technique, the results will always depend on the individual surgeon [12, 13]. Nevertheless the anastomotic technique must be as simple, safe and easily learned as possible. The single-layer continuous technique is being increasingly reported in the literature [2–4], especially since the introduction of the atraumatic, monofil, resorbable suture materials (polyglycolic acid, PDS) [14, 15]. Although the anastomoses which can be performed with single-layer continuous suturing tend to be the easiest ones because they are reversible, these are the most frequently performed in routine clinical practice and are often performed by more junior surgeons. As this technique may be less dependent on the experience of the surgeon and may be easily learned, we decided to introduce this technique to our clinic. After the initial learning phase of 3 months, we started our randomized study. The atraumatic, monofil, double-armed, resorbable 4/0 PDS suture seemed especially suitable for this technique, as it slides easily and without sawing through the tissues. At the beginning of the study some of the more experienced surgeons were concerned about the safety of the technique (Table 2). In the end, however, every surgeon has adopted the new method for all reversible anastomoses, and has extended its indication to include oesophageal and some gastric anastomoses. Using the continuous single-layer colon anastomosis we have also participated in the Swiss Multicenter Trial [16], where within 12 months 586 colonic anastomoses in 545 patients were performed in 22 hospitals. Only two clinical leaks appeared in this series. This study has underlined the safety of the method and convinced all surgeons of the 22 participating hospitals to continue with this technique.

Our clinical experience with the one-layer continuous gastro-intestinal anastomosis convinces us that the technique is non-traumatic, easily learned, safe, simple and quick. Because of the use of only one suture for the anastomosis it is cheaper than other techniques. Because of its simplicity and rapidity, demonstrated in our study of the reversible anastomosis, it is in these cases especially preferable to stapled anastomosis or new techniques such as the biofragmentable ring [17]. It can be recommended for all surgeons, including junior residents in the learning phase and in the future it may be extended to other anastomoses.

References

1. Halsted WS (1887) Circular suture of the intestine: an experimental study. Am J Med Sci 99: 436–461
2. Allen TW, Salem RJ, Stirman JA (1979) Continuous suture for single-layer enteric anastomosis. Texas Surgical Society, Austin, Texas, Oct 1, 1979
3. Bailey HR, LaVoo JW, Max E, Smith KW, Hampton JM (1981) Single-layer continuous colorectal anastomosis. Aust NZ J Surg 51: 473–476
4. Bailey HR, LaVoo JW, Max E, Smith KW, Butts DR, Hampton JM (1984) Single-layer polypropylene colorectal anastomosis – experience with 100 cases. Dis Colon Rectum 27: 19–23
5. Herzog B (1971) Mikroangiographische Studien am Rattendarm zur Prüfung verschiedener Anastomosenarten. Helv Chir Acta 38: 179–184
6. Herzog B (1973) The one-layer and two-layer intestinal anastomosis in animal experiments. Prog Pediatr Surg 5: 37–59
7. Houdart R, Lavergne A, Valleur P, Villet R, Hauteville P (1985) Vascular evolution of single-layer end-on colonic anastomosis. A microangiographic study of 180 anastomoses in the rat from two to 180 days. Dis Colon Rectum 28: 475–480
8. Gambee LP, Garnjobst W, Hardwick CE (1956) Ten years' experience with single-layer anastomosis in colon surgery. Am J Surg 92: 222–227
9. Olsen GB, Letwin E, Williams HT (1968) Clinical experience with the use of a single-layer intestinal anastomosis. Can J Surg 11: 97–100
10. Allgöwer M (1973) Fortschritte der Technik in der Colonchirurgie. Langenbecks Arch Chir 334: 87–98
11. Hell K, Allgöwer M (1976) Die Colonresektion. Springer, Berlin Heidelberg New York
12. Beickert R, von Imhoff C (1984) Nahtinsuffizienz am Dickdarm: ist der Operateur ein Risikofaktor? Chirurg 55: 645–649
13. Seki S (1987) Accuracy of suture placement. Br J Surg 74: 195–197
14. Kull C, Harder F (1986) Die fortlaufende einreihige extramuköse Darmanastomose. Helv Chir Acta 53: 639–642
15. Harder F, Vogelbach P (1988) Single-layer end-on continuous suture of colonic anastomoses. Am J Surg 155: 611–614
16. Vogelbach P, Harder F et al. (1988) Prospektive Erfassungsstudie von 586 konsekutiven fortlaufenden, einreihigen, extramukösen Kolonanastomosen. Helv Chir Acta 55: 655–658
17. Hardy TG, Aguilar PS, Stewart WRC, Katz AR, Maney JW, Costanzo JT, Pace WG (1987) Initial clinical experience with a biofragmentable ring for sutureless bowel anastomosis. Dis Colon Rectum 30: 55–61

Sphincter Preservation in Surgery for Inflammatory Large-Bowel Disease

U. Stoffel and A. Akovbiantz

Recently the therapy of inflammatory large-bowel disease has changed. This is because of several important innovations in the operative treatment and better medical management. Without doubt the pelvic pouch with ileoanal anastomosis procedure after proctocolectomy is of great importance [1, 3, 14, 15, 18]. This continence-preserving operation has been carried out at our clinic since 1987. Based on a review of the literature and our own very limited experience, we will attempt to give some guidelines for the surgical therapy of inflammatory large-bowel disease. The aim of our treatment concept is to give the patient an optimum chance of preserving continence and to improve the results.

Material and Methods

Since 1987, at our hospital ten patients have undergone a pelvic pouch and ileoanal anastomosis procedure with a temporary loop ileostomy. Six patients underwent this operation for ulcerative colitis and four underwent the operation for familial adenomatous polyposis. Two different procedures were performed for ulcerative colitis: a two-stage procedure in three cases and a three-stage procedure in three cases. For familial adenomatous polyposis only, the two-stage procedure was performed.

Pelvic Pouch and Ileoanal Anastomosis (Two-Stage Procedure)

We first carried out a total colectomy with proctomucosectomy followed by fashioning the ileal reservoir and a loop ileostomy. In the second stage we closed the loop ileostomy with a laparotomy and adhesiolysis *par principe* because of the high risk of a postoperative small intestinal obstruction [4, 6, 12].

Pelvic Pouch and Ileoanal Anastomosis (Three-Stage Procedure)

The three-stage procedure consists firstly of a colectomy with preservation of the rectal stump without opening the presacral space or the peritoneum of the pelvic floor and without using a mucous fistula. This is followed by the proctomucosectomy and fashioning of the ileal reservoir with loop ileostomy as the second step and closure of the loop ileostomy with adhesiolysis *par principe* as the third stage.

The indications for a two-stage procedure and a three-stage procedure are described below [13].

Surgical Treatment

We basically distinguish between emergency and elective surgery.

Emergency Surgery

In the case of emergency (e.g. toxic megacolon) we only carry out a colectomy with preservation of the rectal stump and an ileostomy [8, 9, 11, 17]. We do not open the presacral space or the peritoneum of the pelvic floor and we do not use a mucous fistula. This procedure allows the possibility of a later restoration of continuity [9].

Criteria for the Further Procedure. The further procedure depends on histology, clinical follow-up and the state of the rectal stump. Histology plays an essential part as we have seen patients treated for years with a diagnosis of ulcerative colitis who in fact have Crohn's disease [5]. This is of great importance for the choice of therapy to follow. In the case of a histological "unclassified colitis" any further procedure depends on the clinical history. Clinical complications, such as pelvic abscess, ileus or fistula, may also affect further management. Last but not least the state of the rectal stump, fistulae and the function of the sphincter [1] also influence further therapy.

Choice of the Operative Treatment. With a confirmed diagnosis of Crohn's colitis based on histology, clinical follow-up and a disease-free rectal stump we recommend an ileo-rectostomy, although lately the possibility of a pelvic pouch procedure has been discussed as a calculated risk by some authors [1, 2, 5, 8]. With a confirmed diagnosis of ulcerative colitis we carry out a pelvic pouch and ileoanal anastomosis in a three-stage procedure. If the diagnosis

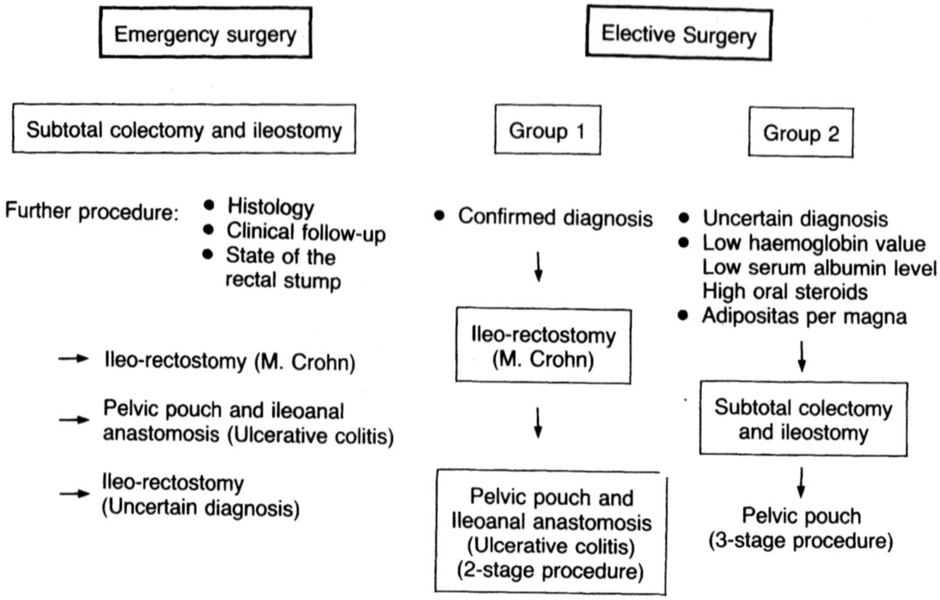

Fig. 1. Criteria and procedures for the surgical therapy of inflammatory large-bowel disease in the case of emergency and elective surgery

is unclear (5%–10%) and the rectal stump free of inflammation the operative treatment is an ileo-rectostomy but if the diagnosis is unclear and the rectal stump involved we leave the ileostomy.

Elective Surgery

In elective surgery we distinguish between two groups: those patients with a confirmed diagnosis, and those patients with an uncertain diagnosis; anaemia; low serum albumin level; patients receiving a high level of oral steroids and patients with adipositas *per magna* [13].

Surgical Treatment (Confirmed Diagnosis) (Group 1). We recommend the ileo-rectostomy for patients with Crohn's disease [8]. For patients with ulcerative colitis the pelvic pouch and ileoanal anastomosis in a two-stage procedure is the therapy of choice.

Surgical Treatment (Risk Group) (Group 2). In patients with an uncertain diagnosis and other risk factors we prefer to carry out a subtotal colectomy with ileostomy as the first step. Any further procedure depends on clinical follow-up and histology. In Crohn's disease we perform an ileo-rectostomy and in ulcerative colitis we carry out the pelvic pouch in a three-stage procedure [13]. If the diagnosis remains unclear after the subtotal colectomy, we temporarily leave the ileostomy.

Conclusions

The pelvic pouch and ileoanal anastomosis as a three-stage procedure is only employed in an emergency, and for those patients with uncertain diagnosis, a high level of oral steroids, anaemia and hypoalbuminaemia and adipositas *per magna* (Fig. 1).

For the ileostomy closure we recommend a laparotomy with adhesiolysis *par principe* because of the high risk of a postoperative small-intestinal obstruction (Fig. 1).

References

1. Beart RW (1988) Proctocolectomy and ileoanal anastomosis. World J Surg 12: 160–163
2. Bloom RJ, Larsen CP, Watt R, Oberhelman HA (1986) A reappraisal of the Kock continent ileostomy in patients with Crohn's disease. Surg Gynecol Obstet 162: 105–108
3. Cohen Z, McLeod RS, Stern H, Grant D, Nordgren S (1985) The pelvic pouch and ileoanal anastamosis procedure. Am J Surg 150: 601–607
4. Dozois RR, Goldberg SM, Rothenberger DA, Utsunomiya J, Nicholls RJ, Cohen Z, Hulten LAG, Moskowitz RL (1986) Restorative proctocolectomy with ileal reservoir. Symposium. Int J Colorectal Dis 1: 2–19
5. Fazio VW, Church JM (1988) Complications and function of the continent ileostomy at the Cleveland Clinic. World J Surg 12: 148–154
6. François Y, Dozois RR, Kelly KA, Beart RW, Wolff BG, Pemberton JH, Ilstrup DM (1989) Small intestinal obstruction complicating ileal pouch-anal anastomosis. Ann Surg 209: 46–50
7. Goligher JC (1988) Surgical treatment of Crohn's disease affecting mainly or entirely the large bowel. World J Surg 12: 186–190
8. Hawley PR (1988) Emergency surgery for ulcerative colitis. World J Surg 12: 169–173
9. Morel P, Hawker PC, Allan RN, Dykes PW, Alexander-Williams J (1986) Management of acute colitis in inflammatory bowel disease. World J Surg 10: 814–819
10. Mortensen N (1988) Progress with the pouch – restorative proctocolectomy for ulcerative colitis. Gut 29: 561–565
11. Nicholls RJ, Holt SDH, Lubowski DZ (1989) Restorative proctocolectomy with ileal reservoir. Comparison of two-stage vs. three-stage procedures and analysis of factors that might affect outcome. Dis Colon Rectum 32: 323–326
12. Parks AG, Nicholls RJ, Belliveau P (1980) Proctocolectomy with ileal reservoir and anal anastomosis. Br J Surg 67: 533–538
13. Rothenberger DA, Vermeulen FD, Christenson Ce, Balcos EG, Nemer FD, Goldberg SM, Bellirean P, Nivatvongs S, Schotten JL, Fang DT, Kennedy HL (1983) Restorative proctocolectomy with ileal reservoir and ileoanal anastomosis. Am J Surg 145: 82–88

14. Scott NA, Dozois RR, Beart RW, Pemberton JH, Wolff BG, Ilstrup DM (1988) Postoperative intra-abdominal and pelvic sepsis complicating ileal pouch-anal anastomosis. Int J Colorectal Dis 3: 149–152
15. Truelove SC, Marks CG (1981) Toxic megacolon part I: pathogenesis, diagnosis and treatment. Clin Gastroenterol 10: 107–117
16. Utsunomiya T, Iwama M, Imajo M, Matsuo A, Sawai S, Yaegashi K, Hirayama R (1980) Total colectomy, mucosal proctectomy and ileoanal anastomosis. Dis Colon Rectum 23: 459–466

Critical Appraisal of Hartmann's Operation for Rectosigmoid Surgical Emergencies

C.A. Cabre-Martinez, C. Ballesta-Lopez, B. Nieto-Martinez and A. Osorio-Gullon

Introduction

Inflammatory, neoplastic or traumatic lesions of the sigmoid colon or rectum may present acutely as low intestinal obstruction, perforation with peritonitis, or severe bleeding. Conservative methods of treatment often carry a high mortality [1–3]; surgeons in recent years have opted for more aggressive methods of treatment [4–9] such as emergency resection of the affected bowel, sometimes followed by primary anastomosis [7], with or without a protective proximal colostomy, or by iliac end-colostomy: in these cases the distal stump may be closed by suturing (Hartmann's operation) [8, 9] or may be brought to the surface as a mucous fistula.

None of these techniques is free from complications, but the reported results are better than those obtained by more conservative surgical methods [3, 5–8] particularly when peritoneal contamination is present. A 15-year experience with Hartmann's operation for such problems forms the basis of the present study, the results of which are critically analysed.

Patients

Seventy-three patients who were suffering from an acute abdomen due to inflammatory, traumatic or malignant disease of the sigmoid colon or rectum were operated on as an emergency.

Sex and Age. Thirty-five patients were men and 38 women. Their ages ranged between 21 and 85 years, with 47 of them (64.3%) over the age of 60 and 26 (35.6%) in the 70–85 year range.

Aetiology. Fifty patients suffered from carcinoma (18 men and 32 women), 21 had complicated diverticular disease (17 men and 4 women), one young woman had a traumatic perforation of her sigmoid colon and one elderly man a sigmoid perforation due to ischaemia.

Clinical Presentation. Forty patients had obstruction, all but one being due to carcinoma. Thirty-two presented with peritonitis on admission. In 20 this was due to diverticular disease, in 10 it complicated an obstructing carcinoma and in the other two patients it was due to trauma and ischaemia. Severe bleeding from a non-obstructing carcinoma of the sigmoid colon occurred in one patient. Ten patients were in shock on admission, eight of whom had peritonitis. The other two had large-bowel obstruction due to carcinoma, but no peritonitis.

A high incidence of associated diseases was present in the over 60 year old group: seven patients had chronic respiratory problems (one of them on long-term steroid therapy), six had cardiovascular disease, and three had metabolic diseases (diabetes mellitus, chronic renal failure, and chronic renal failure plus liver cirrhosis). One patient had polyposis.

Methods

Standard investigations and resuscitation were carried out as an emergency. Bowel preparation was not carried out in any patient. All patients were operated on as an emergency. A mid-line laparotomy incision was made. If pus was present, specimens were sent for aerobic and anaerobic culture and sensitivity. The diseased bowel was isolated, and excised. Normally the retrorectal space was not extensively dissected, unless it was necessary for excision of the disease or for abscess drainage. In the case of carcinoma without distant metastases or gross local spread, and provided the patient's general condition allowed, a radical resection was performed. The distal rectal stump was sutured with fine non-absorbable stitches and left in the pelvic cavity. Peritoneal lavage was carried out at the end of the procedure with copious warm 0.9% NaCl solution, sometimes with added antibiotics or Betadine.

A proximal end-colostomy was performed in the left lower quadrant. The pelvic cavity was drained via separate stab incisions. The laparotomy wound was sutured with interrupted stitches, with tension sutures in some patients. More recently, the skin has initially been left unsutured in patients with peritoneal contamination; it is then sutured after a few days.

Results

Mortality. Eight patients died in the postoperative period (11%). Five of them had an obstructing carcinoma; three had shock on admission, due in

Table 1. Postoperative complications

Complication		No. of cases
Wound infection		19
Abdominal wound dehiscence		2
Intra-abdominal abscess		5
Colostomy complications		6
Early		
Ischaemic necrosis	1	
Peri-colostomy abscess	1	
Late		
Stenosis	1	
Prolapse	2	
Retraction	1	
Small-bowel obstruction due to adhesions		1
Respiratory complications		9
Deep venous thrombosis		2
Cerebro-vascular accident		1
Transient renal failure		2
Bleeding duodenal ulcer		1
Incisional hernia		5

two cases to faecal peritonitis. The other three patients who died had perforated sigmoid diverticular disease with localised peritonitis; two of them had septic shock.

These patients died from intra-abdominal or respiratory sepsis, or a combination of both: two, with chronic renal failure, developed acute renal failure. The mortality for complicated acute diverticulitis was 14% and for all types of peritonitis 16%. Patients who were in shock on admission had a 50% mortality, whether they had peritonitis or not.

Morbidity. Postoperative complications occurred in 35 of the 65 patients who survived the operation; these are summarised in Table 1. Five patients developed incisional hernia as a late complication.

Reconstructive Procedures. Restoration of intestinal continuity was attempted in 34 of 65 patients who survived the operation, after an average delay of 6.8 months. A colorectal anastomosis was performed in 29 patients, a total colectomy and ileorectal anastomosis in one, and an abdominoperineal excision of rectum also in one. Five of the carcinoma patients had tumour spread at this second operation, and in three of them no reconstructive procedure was carried out. The other 31 were not operated on mainly because they were satisfied with their colostomy or because of old age, poor health or signs of advancing carcinoma.

Discussion

Data available from the literature show that the acute abdomen in patients with a pathological process of left colon or rectum carries a high mortality when conservative surgical procedures are employed. Botsford et al. [1] report 100% mortality in 11 patients with colon perforation treated by suture, drainage and diverting colostomy, while Brown and Toomey [2], Liebert and DeWeese [5] and Madden and Tan [7] report mortality rates between 39% and 46% for patients surgically treated by anything less than resection of the diseased bowel. A fistula may occur despite an adequate diverting colostomy in patients with acute diverticulitis [5].

Resection of the affected bowel in the acute stage has the advantage that it removes the septic focus, the continuing source of contamination, and, if present, resolves the obstruction. Primary anastomosis is contraindicated because the bowel is unprepared, distended, oedematous and often surrounded by bacterial contamination [7, 8, 10]. When a proximal end-colostomy is formed, the distal end of the bowel may be oversewn, or a mucous fistula constructed. This may not be easy to achieve, though, in the presence of inflammation, oedema, and thickening of the mesocolon such as occurs in diverticular disease.

Conclusions

Hartmann's operation is a useful procedure, but it has its limitations!

References

1. Botsford TW, Zollinger RM, Hicks R (1971) Mortality of the surgical treatment of diverticulitis. Am J Surg 121: 702–705
2. Brown DB, Toomey WF (1960) Diverticular disease of the colon. A review of 258 cases. Br J Surg 47: 485–493
3. Crile GJr (1954) Danger of conservative surgery in abdominal emergencies. Surgery 35: 122
4. Gallagher DM, Russell TR (1978) Surgical management of diverticular disease. Surg Clin North Am 58: 563–572
5. Liebert CW, DeWeese BM (1981) Primary resection without anastomosis for perforation of acute diverticulitis. Surg Gynecol Obstet 152: 30–32
6. Lubbers EJC, De Boer HHM (1982) Inherent complications of Hartmann's operation. Surg Gynecol Obstet 155: 717–721
7. Madden JL, Tan PY (1961) Primary resection and anastomosis in the treatment of perforated lesions of the colon, with abscess or diffusing peritonitis. Surg Gynecol Obstet 113: 646–650

8. ReMine SG, Dozois RR (1981) Hartmann's procedure: its use with complicated carcinomas of sigmoid colon and rectum. Arch Surg 116: 630–633
9. Sames CP (1960) Resection of carcinoma of the colon in the presence of obstruction. Lancet 3: 948–949
10. Kuhlmayer R (1981) Causes of suture dehiscence in colorectal surgery. Coloproctology 3: 15–16

Endoanal Surgical Repair of Rectocoele

M.-C. MARTI

Introduction

Very little attention has been given to the problem of rectocoeles. Their symptoms and clinical manifestations resulting from herniation of the anterior rectal wall have been underestimated by gynaecologists, surgeons and gastro-enterologists. Rectocoeles should be differentiated from enterocoeles.

Rectocoele develops by definition only in the middle third of the vagina. At this level, the posterior vaginal wall becomes thinner. The weakness and attenuation of the central fibrous perineal body contributes to the formation of an anterior suprasphincteric pocket. As the rectal wall has a great distensibility, it is stretched and the resulting pocket of rectal mucosa protrudes through the dehiscence of the musculo-fascial vaginal septum. The internal and external sphincter and the levators represent a relatively fixed block. With increasing weakness of the perineal body and the rectovaginal fascia, the defect moves inferiorly and anteriorly relative to the sphincter. Any further straining will push stools further from the anal opening. The size and position of the pocket can explain the various symptoms associated with rectocoele.

Symptoms

It is difficult to distinguish symptoms due to a rectocoele from those due to complications of a rectocoele and from those produced by associated lesions. Furthermore, it is impossible to correlate symptoms with severity of the rectocoele.

Most frequently associated symptoms are rectal fullness, perception of a perineal mass, incomplete evacuation, protrusion, pain, bleeding and soiling. Urge to defaecate is normal but the patient "can't get it out"; faeces seems to stick near the opening. A more or less severe anorectal outlet obstruction may develop. Patients have to support the posterior vaginal wall digitally to pass stools. Of the 50 patients reported by Capps, 76% suffered from constipation and 39% used manual assistance [1].

During straining, a rectocoele becomes full of faeces and interferes with emptying of the rectum. Repeated straining results in mucosal prolapse complicated by more or less extensive proctitis and intussusception of the anterior part of the rectum. This produces a valve mechanism which is responsible for some of the major symptoms: the prolapse obstruction or "roll-down" syndrome described by Sullivan [8].

In cases of associated descending perineum in cases where the external sphincter has been damaged previously, incontinence may develop. Patients complain of incomplete and uncontrolled evacuation with faecal soiling.

Contraction of the puborectalis sling results in an anterior retraction of the anal canal but the laxity of the anterior wall prevents obliteration of the anorectal lumen. In a paradoxic manner, the more the patient contracts the puborectalis muscle, the more he or she loses some faeces. Subsequent vigorous cleaning of the perineum may increase the mucosal prolapse and produce anodermal excoriation.

A rectocoele is therefore associated with symptoms which may be caused by the rectocoele alone or it may be associated with various other anorectal lesions producing pain, bleeding, prolapse and constipation. It may be associated with lesions according to the weakness of the various perineal structures:

- Descending perineum
- Haemorrhoids
- Mucosal prolapse
- Solitary rectal ulcer
- Intussusception
- Uterine prolapse
- Cystocoele
- Faecal incontinence and soiling
- Urinary incontinence

A rectocoele may be complicated by bleeding due to ischaemia and resulting ulceration and by rectovaginal fistula.

There is a natural reticence by patients to discuss their problems and how they handle them. Precise questions must be addressed. As reported by Khubchandani they may respond as follows [2]:

- "I don't seem to be able to empty myself".
- "I feel constant pressure down there".
- "There is a bearing-down sensation".
- "I have to use a syringe or an enema to empty myself".
- "I have to use pressure around the rectum".
- "I have to use my fingers in the vagina or the rectum".
- "There is a sensation of a pouch or a hernia down there".

Diagnosis

The diagnosis is essentially established by clinical examination. A hooked finger is pressed in the anterior rectal wall to detect the weakness of the septum. Bimanual examination is necessary to exclude associated lesions. Defaecography confirms the diagnosis.

Treatment

Surgery is the only way to treat a rectocoele definitively. Patients with severe constipation should be treated initially by dietary manipulation and bulk laxatives. If clinical manifestations are not improved after a few weeks, surgery should be offered. Biofeedback is useful only if evidence of anism has been established.

Several questions are raised by surgical treatment: should a rectocoele be repaired through a vaginal approach or should it be corrected through an endorectal route? Should other associated anorectal lesions be repaired simultaneously and when and how should urogenital prolapse be corrected?

A colpoperineorrhaphy with resection of the sac or vaginal herniorrhaphy alone is insufficient. Colpocleisis with or without Mersilene mesh reinforcement to reduce an enterocoele should be reserved for a small number of elderly patients where there is no requirement to preserve sexual function.

A rectocoele complicated by incontinence may be best treated by an extensive posterior colpomyorrhaphy with sphincter reconstruction. Such a posterior colpomyorrhaphy may be difficult to perform; lateral structures are retracted and loose. Narrowing should be prevented. Several complications may occur: delayed healing, suture line dehiscence, rectovaginal fistula in the case of too deeply placed sutures, haematoma, infection, insufficiency of sphincter repair and postoperative dyspareunia. Furthermore, the reduction of the rectocoele results in a prolapse of the rectal mucosa responsible for the roll-down syndrome and bleeding.

According to Redding [5], Marks [3], Sehapayak [7], Capps [1], Sullivan [8] and Sarles [5], transvaginal repair of the rectocoele will not provide sufficient relief. These authors developed a combined rectovaginal approach or even a purely endorectal technique of repair. A purely endorectal approach allows simultaneous correction of any anorectal pathologic findings.

The patient may be operated on in the jack-knife or lithotomy position. We prefer lithotomy position. The rectum should be emptied with laxatives or enemas. General anaesthesia, peridural block, spinal anaesthesia, caudal block or even extensive local anaesthesia may be used. A short course of systemic broad spectrum antibiotics is given. A Sims, a Hill-Fergusson or a Park's anal retractor is inserted. The length of the rectovaginal septum defect is checked digitally. The submucosa is infiltrated with saline. A 3-cm transverse slightly curved incision is made above the dentate line or just below the upper extremity of the anterior anal canal. The submucosal plane is dissected as far as the point which has been palpated above the weakness of the septum. Haemostasis is performed step-by-step. The curved incision may be increased by vertical incisions on each end of the transverse one. The lax rectovaginal septum is closed by separate transverse stitches of 3-0 polyglycolic acid sutures.

According to Khubchandani, transverse sutures plicating the septum are placed first [2]. Sutures are placed 1 cm apart from outside inward. Stitches approximate the puborectalis muscle and also the rectovaginal fascia 3–4 cm above it. Two or three vertical sutures of the same material are placed between the proximal and distal points plicating the rectovaginal septum like a venetian curtain and shortening the anterior rectal wall. According to Sarles, if there is no incontinence, the vertical sutures are sufficient [6]. As in Delormes's procedure for rectal prolapse, the rectovaginal septum is reinforced by plication. Any excess of mucosa is excised and the wound closed by interrupted sutures of 3-0 Dexon or chromic catgut.

The vertical plicating sutures initially recommended by Sullivan [8] and later by Khubchandani [2] and Sarles [6] allow mucosal resection, leaving short and viable flaps which can be sutured without tension. This reduces the risk of flap retraction, mucosal sloughing and delayed healing.

Packing is usually unnecessary. We use a rectal tube wrapped with Tabotam for 24 h to ensure good adhesion of the mucosa to the underlying structures and to prevent haematoma formation. Early postoperative bowel movement is encouraged with laxatives and mucilages. Sitz baths are useless. Postoperative pain may be prevented with 100 mg Voltarene per day.

Any concomitant anorectal lesion may be treated simultaneously: haemorrhoids, tags, and fissures may be excised. Hypertonia of the internal sphincter in cases of recurrent fissure may be treated by submucosal sphincterotomy. The only disadvantage of the anorectal approach is that it does not offer simultaneous correction of a cystocoele.

We have treated 33 women aged between 34 and 78 years. Twenty-five of them were uni- or multiparous; 12 out of 25 were multiparous. Symptoms were present from 1 to 30 years. Eighteen complained of constipation and 12 of incontinence. Three presented a solitary rectal ulcer within the rectocoele. Perineal descent was present in 26 women. The anal canal had a very important asymmetrical length in 11 women. Ten short anterior anal canals were present among the 12 women suffering from incontinence. A short anterior anal canal was present in only 1 among 18 patients suffering from constipation. Previous perineal surgery had been performed on 21 patients. Hysterectomy, cystopexy and rectopexy were among the most frequently performed procedures. Transverse plication completed by longitudinal plication was performed on 12 patients suffering from incontinence

Table 1. Published data on surgical repair of rectocoele

Authors	No. of patients	Follow-up (years)	Success rate (%)
Sullivan [8]	151	1.5	79.5
Capps [1]	51	NK	94.0
Sehapayak [7]	355	NK	84.5
Khubchandani [2]	59	1.5	80.0
Sarles [6]	20	3	95.0
Marti [4]	33	1	90.0

NK, not known

and presenting a short anterior anal canal. Longitudinal plication alone was performed in 21 cases.

There was no postoperative morbidity or mortality. The hospital stay was less than 4 days in each instance.

Functional results were very good. Eleven out of 12 patients suffering from incontinence associated with rectocoele were cured. In the one remaining case, the degree of incontinence was reduced.

Nine out of 21 cases suffering from constipation had spontaneous and normal evacuation after surgery; two patients still required laxatives. These results compare favourably with previous published data from the literature (Table 1).

In our experience, rectocoele associated with a short anterior anal canal can be well treated by a transanal approach. Rectocoele with sphincter rupture should, as before, be treated by posterior colpomyorrhaphy.

Conclusion

The endoanal approach to rectocoele seems to give far better results than any other surgical approach in managing such a distressing lesion.

References

1. Capps WF (1975) Rectoplasty and perineoplasty for the symptomatic rectocele. A report of fifty cases. Dis Colon Rectum 18: 237–244
2. Khubchandani IT, Sheets JA, Stasik JJ, Hakki AR (1983) Endorectal repair of rectocele. Dis Colon Rectum 26: 792–796
3. Marks MM (1967) The rectal side of the rectocele. Dis Colon Rectum 10: 387–388
4. Marti M-C (1989) Les rectocèles. Ann Gastroenterol Hepatol 25: 309–311
5. Redding MD (1965) The relaxed perineum and anorectal disease. Dis Colon Rectum 8: 279–282

6. Sarles JC, Arnaud A, Selezneff I, Olivier S (1989) Endo-rectal repair of rectocele. Int J Colorectal Dis 4: 167–171
7. Sehapayak S (1985) Transrectal repair of rectocele. An extended armamentarium of colorectal surgeons. A report of 355 cases. Dis Colon Rectum 28: 422–433
8. Sullivan ES, Leaverton GH, Hardwick CE (1968) Transrectal perineal repair: an adjunct to improved function after anorectal surgery. Dis Colon Rectum 11: 106–114

Excision and Primary Closure or Excision and Secondary Healing in the Treatment of Natal Cleft Sinus: A Prospective Study

H.T. KHAWAJA and P.C. WEAVER

Introduction

The first reported case of a successfully treated pilonidal sinus was described by Anderson in 1847 [1]. Since then, numerous procedures have been used to treat this pathology. They run the gamut from simple injection of phenol [2] to radical excision of the affected area with or without primary closure [3–6], including Z-plasty and lumbar rotation flaps to close the defect [7]. This multiplicity of surgical techniques, together with reported recurrence rates varying from 1% to 43% [5, 6], are testimony to the morbidity of the disease and the inefficacy of its treatment.

This study was undertaken to evaluate two commonly used methods of treatment of natal cleft sinus: excision and primary closure and excision and healing by secondary intention.

Patients and Methods

All patients between 16 and 60 years of age, with symptomatic natal cleft sinus, were considered. Patients with lesions associated with cellulitis or abscess formation were excluded from the trial and treated by excision and healing by granulation. Patients suffering from diabetus mellitus, those on steroids and those judged unsuitable for day case surgery were not considered. All patients gave informed consent.

Over a period of 49 months, 46 consecutive patients entered the trial and were randomly allocated to two treatment groups: excision and primary closure and excision and secondary healing. All procedures were done under general anaesthetic with the patient in the jack-knife position and the buttocks held apart with adhesive strapping. Wide shaving of the area was carried out, especially deep in the natal cleft. In an attempt to achieve total excision, pits were injected with methylene blue using a 20-g Teflon cannula after removing its metal introducer. Special care was taken not to inject under pressure or to probe sinus tracts in order to avoid staining of normal tissue and wider excision than necessary. In all cases, an ellipse of skin, encompassing all the pits, and subcutaneous tissue was sharply excised down to the presacral fascia. Special care was taken not to undermine the lateral edges of resection. Haemostasis was achieved by diathermy.

For excision and healing by granulation, the cavity was packed with gauze soaked in aqueous proflavine. The pack was changed daily and the patient allowed home when packing was tolerable without parenteral analgesia. Primary closure was achieved using Prolene deep mattress sutures placed 2 cm apart, after releasing the strapping holding the buttocks apart. Mobility of skin and subcutaneous tissue over the sacrum was maintained by avoiding the placement of sutures in the presacral fascia. The patients were discharged home with a supply of oral analgesic tablets (Co-dydramol tablets containing dihydrocodeine tartrate 10 mg and paracetamol 500 mg). The operative site, in both groups, was infiltrated with 10 ml of 0.25% bupivacaine with adrenaline 1 in 200 000.

All patients were given strict hygiene instructions and were reviewed weekly until healing occurred and also at 6 and 12 months postoperatively. Healing was defined as complete epithelisation of the operative site. In the secondary healing group, the proflavine pack was changed daily for the first week; then, on the first out-patient visit, it was replaced by a silicone foam which was renewed weekly until healing occurred. In the primary closure group, the sutures were removed on the 14th postoperative day or earlier in the case of patient discomfort. If healing by primary closure failed, the wound was then allowed to heal by granulation.

Chi-squared tests with Yates correction and Mann-Whitney U tests were used for between group comparison.

Results

There was no between group difference in the age and sex distribution of patients (Table 1). The number of pits associated with the natal cleft sinus were similar in both treatment groups (Table 1). In the excision and secondary healing group, all patients had successful treatment as defined by complete healing of the wound, and there were no recorded complications. In the primary closure group, there were no complications in 74% of cases

Table 1. Comparability of groups

	Sex		Age		Number of pits	
	Male	Female	Median	Range	Median	Range
Primary closure	19	4	25	19–45	2	1–5
Secondary healing	17	6	23	16–47	2	1–4

(17 out of 23) and the wound remained healed after removal of sutures. However, the treatment failed in 26% of cases (6 out of 23). The wound broke open in four patients after removal of sutures. These patients had no evidence of cellulitis or wound discharge. However, bacteriological swab and culture, immediately after removal of sutures, grew both aerobic and anaerobic organisms in three of the four cases. Two patients required early unscheduled follow-up because of pain, and underwent premature removal of sutures on the second postoperative day for wound haematoma and ninth postoperative day for wound infection. The patient with haematoma was admitted for 1 day and required general anaesthetic to evacuate the clots, clean the wound, and check the haemostasis. All failed cases were converted to treatment by secondary healing.

All patients in the primary closure group underwent day case surgery. One patient with haematoma required readmission for another day. The median hospital stay in the secondary healing group was 3 days (range, 2–3 days; Table 2). For those patients treated successfully by primary closure, the wound remained healed after removal of sutures on the 14th postoperative day. This time was significantly less than the time taken to healing in the secondary healing group: a median of 41 days (range = 29–51 days; Table 2). However, for the failed cases in the primary closure group who were converted to treatment by secondary healing, the time to healing (median, 37.5; range, 26–48 days) was not significantly different from that of the secondary healing group (Table 2).

Patients successfully treated by primary closure had a shorter time off work (median, 17; range, 15–21 days) compared to the secondary healing group (median, 42; range, 28–56 days; Table 2). However, there was no difference in the time off work between the failed primary closure subgroup (median, 38.5; range, 28–49 days) and the secondary healing group (median, 42; range, 28–56 days; Table 2). Seventeen per cent of patients treated by primary closure (4 out of 23) were dissatisfied with their

Table 2. Clinical data

	Primary closure group				Secondary healing group	
	Success (n = 17)		Failure (n = 6)			
	Median	Range	Median	Range	Median	Range
Days in hospital	1 (day case)*		1	1–2*	3	2–3
Days to healing	14 (removal of sutures)*		37.5	26–48[a]	41	29–51
Days off work	17	15–21*	38.5	28–49[a]	42	28–56

*$p < 0.001$
[a] Not significant vs secondary healing group

treatment compared to 65% of patients (15 out of 23) treated by secondary healing, who required regular outpatient attendance and longer time off work.

There was no evidence of recurrence in either groups at 6 and 12 months follow-up. One patient who failed to heal in the primary closure group was lost to follow up at 12 months. She was a final year student at the local polytechnic college and had moved out of the catchment area.

Discussion

The ideal treatment for natal cleft sinus should give quick healing and a low recurrence rate while avoiding hospital stay, and minimising patient inconvenience and time off work. This prospective randomized study has shown that successful day case excision and primary closure of natal cleft sinus is feasible and offers earlier healing and return to work compared to excision and healing by secondary intention. Although the failure rate is high (26%), the hospital stay is shorter, and the time to complete healing and return to work for the failed primary closure patients is not significantly different to that of the secondary healing group.

The failure rate in the primary closure group is higher than that reported in the literature for a similar technique [8]. Four of the six patients who failed to heal had bacteriological evidence of an infected wound which may have been the main cause of the high failure rate in the primary closure group. Kronborg et al. [9] have reported that the prophylactic use of clindamycin reduced healing time after primary closure. None of our patients received prophylactic antibiotics.

Patients' dissatisfaction with the treatment received was taken as a measure of their inconvenience. Primary closure caused less dissatisfaction than secondary healing.

A possible criticism of this study would be that the operation of excision and secondary healing was not carried out as a day case. Attempts to send these patients home the same day, prior to the present study, failed as patients reported intolerable pain and both hospital and district nurses strongly felt that parenteral as opposed to oral analgesia would be required to change the pack for the first 2–3 days.

Our patients were followed up for 12 months only; recurrences over longer periods of time have, however, been reported [8]. Natal cleft sinus affects mainly the young [4] who, in the south of England, are frequently on the move and therefore longer follow-up would be difficult.

This study demonstrates that excision and primary closure of uncomplicated natal cleft sinus is preferable to the conventional excision and secondary healing and is likely to generate huge savings, not only in terms of health care resources but also in lost income due to time off work. Further studies are needed to compare excision and primary closure to other proven methods of treatment which do not require hospitalisation.

References

1. Anderson AW (1847) Hair extracted from an ulcer. Bost Med Surg J 36: 74
2. Stansby G, Greatorex R (1989) Phenol treatment of pilonidal sinuses of the natal cleft. Br J Surg 76: 729–730
3. Goodall P (1961) The aetiology and treatment of pilonidal sinus. A review of 163 patients. Br J Surg 49: 212–218
4. Clothier PR, Haywood IR (1984) The natural history of post anal (pilonidal) sinus. Ann R Coll Surg Engl 66: 201–203
5. Wood RAB, Williams RHP, Hughes LE (1977) Foam elastomer dressing in the management of open granulating wounds: experience with 250 patients. Br J Surg 64: 554–557
6. Sood SC, Green JR, Parui R (1975) Results of various operations for sacrococcygeal pilonidal disease. Plast Reconstr Surg 56: 559–566
7. Lamke LO, Larsson J, Nylen B (1979) Treatment of pilonidal sinus by radical excision and reconstruction by rotation flap surgery or Z-plasty technique. Scand J Plast Reconstr Surg 13: 351–353
8. Allen-Mersh TG (1990) Pilonidal sinus: finding the right track for treatment. Br J Surg 77: 123–132
9. Kronborg O, Christensen K, Zimmermann-Nielsen C (1985) Chronic pilonidal disease: a randomized trial with a complete 3-year follow-up. Br J Surg 72: 303–304

Part II: Cancer

Prognostic Value of Dukes and Jass Classifications of Colorectal Cancer

E.P. SARAGA, N. DE QUAY, J.-C. GIVEL and X. ALBE

Introduction

In an attempt to improve the prognostic accuracy for colon carcinoma, numerous alternative classifications have been proposed [1–13].

In 1932 Cuthbert Dukes proposed a pathological staging [2] based on the depth of penetration of the tumour through the bowel wall and the presence or absence of lymph node metastases in the resected specimen. The method has been modified [4], clinical information about curability has been added and the D stage has been introduced [14]. The Dukes system is one of the most widely used classifications and its prognostic value well established.

In 1986 J.R. Jass proposed a new prognostic system for rectal cancer [15–17]. His grading system was constructed using the Cox regression model [18]. Four variables were selected in the best model [16]: the extent of spread through the bowel wall, the number of affected lymph nodes, the pattern of tumour growth (expanding/infiltrating) and the peritumoral lymphocytic infiltration.

The aim of this study was to compare the prognostic value of the Jass and Dukes classifications after extending the first to the entire colon and to appreciate the possible advantages of using the two classifications together.

Materials and Methods

For this study we selected patients who fulfilled the following criteria:

1. First occurrence of large bowel carcinoma excluding the synchronous cancers
2. Sporadic type of disease (carcinoma arising in familial adenomatous polyposis, in cancer family syndromes or in chronic inflammatory idiopathic colitis were excluded)
3. Curative tumour resection (no evidence at the time of laparotomy of distant spread or of residual cancer)

Table 1. Follow-up of patients

Follow-up	Procedure
Every 3 months	Clinical examination, carcinoembryonic antigen, haemoglobin, leucocytes, ALP, SR
Every 6 months	Sigmoidoscopy
Every 12 months	Chest X-ray, colonoscopy
In particular cases	Ultrasound of the liver, abdominal and thoracic CT, immunoscintigraphy

ALP, alkaline phosphatase; SR, sedimentation rate; CT, computed tomography

Between January 1985 and December 1986, 215 patients with a histological diagnosis of adenocarcinoma of the colon or rectum had a resection in the Surgical Department of the University Hospital of Lausanne Medical School or of the Hospital of Sion (Valais). Of these 215 patients 171 fulfilled the criteria stated previously. These 171 patients were part of a continuing prospective study of large-bowel cancer and follow-up was completed on every patient to the end of 1989. The protocol used for the follow-up is summarised in Table 1. At each assessment patients were classified into one of the following groups: (a) without sign of recurrence, (b) suspected recurrence, (c) confirmed recurrence and (d) death (related or unrelated to the carcinoma).

Patients who died within 30 days of surgery and those whose follow-up data were judged insufficient were excluded from the analysis. Also excluded from the survival analysis were the patients whose death was not related to the colonic carcinoma. Only deaths due to carcinoma were included. The survival data were finally analysed for a group of 144 patients.

All histological slides were reviewed and the following histopathological variables were considered:

Type of Tumour. Tumours were classified as adenocarcinoma, mucinous carcinoma or signet-ring cell carcinoma according to WHO criteria [19].

Overall Differentiation. Tumours were graded as poorly, moderately or well-differentiated according to the guidelines of Dukes and Bussey [4].

Pattern of Growth. Tumours were divided into expanding and infiltrating as recommended by Ming for gastric carcinoma [20].

Lymphocytic Infiltration. This was assessed at the advancing front of the tumour, based on the "worst" area following the J.R. Jass description [15] and graded as positive or negative.

Lymphatic, blood vessel, and perineural invasion was searched for. The presence of vascular invasion was confirmed by elastic tissue stains when indicated [21].

Results

Age and Sex of Patients

The age span for the series was between 36 and 96 years with an average age of 71 years. There were 82 females and 77 males.

Tumour Characteristics

The location of the tumours was: 14 caecum (9%), 17 ascending colon (11%), 13 transverse colon (8.5%), 15 descending colon (9.3%), 37 sigmoid (23.4%) and 62 rectum (39%). The tumours measured in their maximal axis between 1 and 10 cm (5 cm average). Of all cases 41% measured more than 5 cm and 11% were 3 cm or less. There were 150 (93.8%) adenocarcinomas, 18 (11%) mucinous carcinomas and only 2 (1.2%) signeting cell carcinomas. No particular feature was related to location, age or sex.

Jass and Dukes Classifications

The distribution of the 144 cases according to the Dukes and Jass classifications and the survival results are shown in Fig. 1.

The distribution of patients according to both systems of classification is presented in Table 2 and the number of deaths in each subgroup in Fig. 2.

Figure 3 shows the increase in the proportion of deaths inside the Dukes B group of patients in relation to the Jass prognostic groups. There was a 10% death rate in the Dukes B–Jass I patients, 20% in the Dukes B–Jass II patients and 40% in the Dukes B–Jass III patients.

Two other factors were important for survival in our study: vascular invasion and the degree of differentiation of the tumour (Figs. 4, 5).

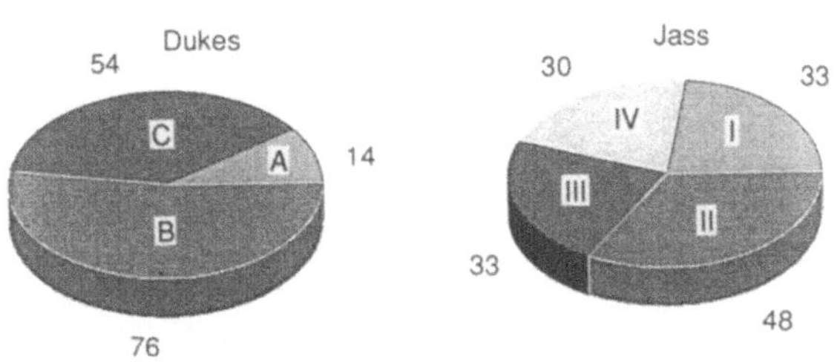

Fig. 1. Distribution and survival of 144 patients with curative surgery 1983–1985. Survival: Dukes A = 100%, B = 76.3%, C = 55.5%. Jass I = 93.9%, II = 75.0%, III = 57.5%, IV = 53.3%

Table 2. Distribution of 144 patients according to Jass and Dukes classifications

	Jass I	Jass II	Jass III	Jass IV
Dukes A	12	2	0	0
Dukes B	20	34	22	0
Dukes C	1	12	11	30

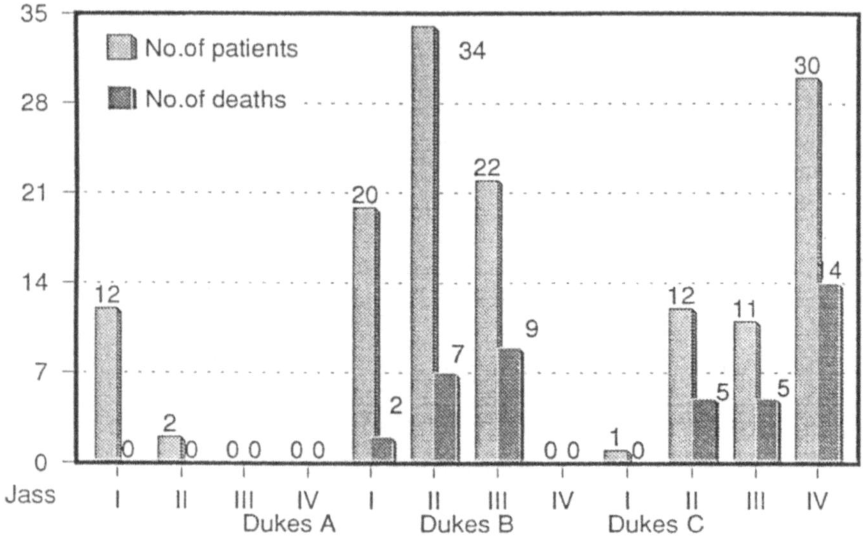

Fig. 2. Distribution of 144 patients with curative surgery according to Jass and Dukes classifications showing number of deaths in each subgroup

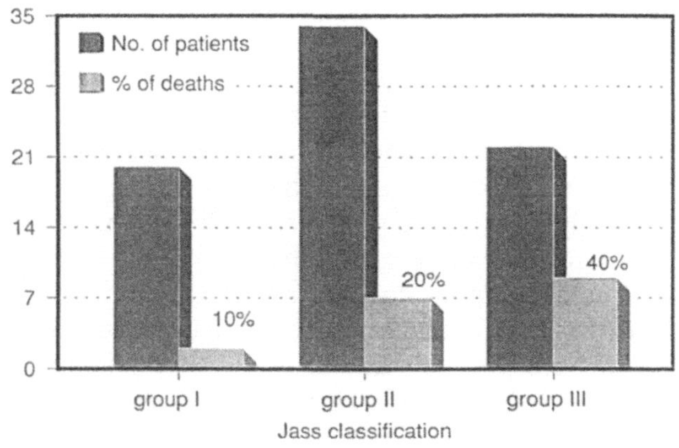

Fig. 3. Proportion of deaths in the Dukes B group of 76 patients in relation to Jass groups

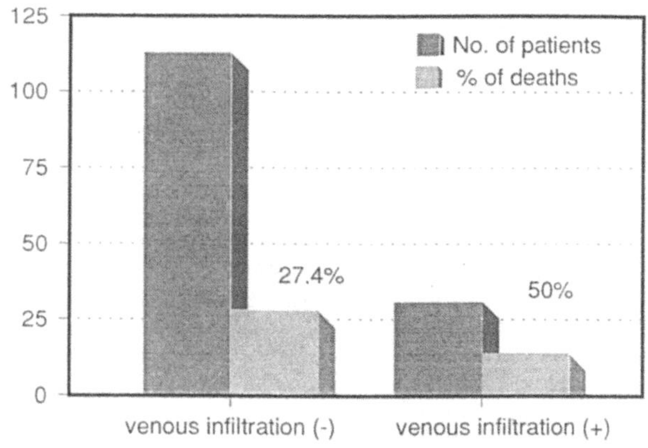

Fig. 4. Tumoral venous infiltration

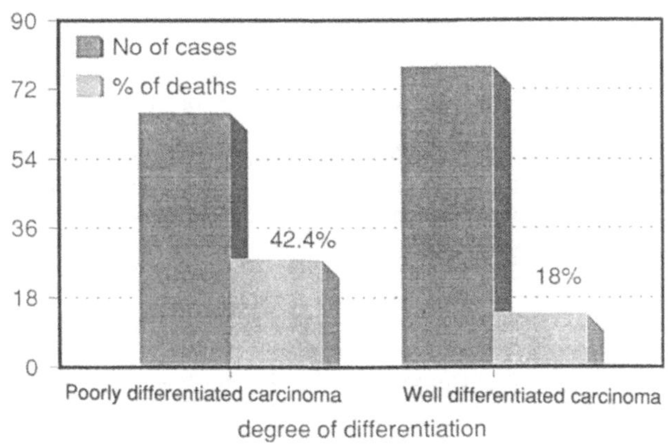

Fig. 5. Differentiation of the carcinoma

Discussion

As in Jass's original study, the distribution of our patients constituted four groups of approximately equal size, whereas in the Dukes classification more than 50% of the patients were in the B stage. Survival figures generally confirm the prognostic value of the Jass classification; however, it is of note that in our study there is not a great difference between survival data concerning the Jass groups III and IV which both had a fair prognosis. This is perhaps related to the relatively short time of the follow-up, limited for this prospective study to only 3–4 years. The most interesting observation was the fact that the simultaneous use of the two classifications allowed a stratification of patients inside the Dukes B group into 3 subgroups with clear prognostic differences. Our data suggest that it may be perhaps of value to offer in selected cases, such as the Dukes B–Jass III group of patients, an adjuvant therapy aimed at eradicating occult disease. To conclude, in our opinion the scoring system proposed by Jass is simple, reproducible and improves the prognostic assessment of colorectal cancer.

References

1. Lockhart-Mummery JP (1926) Two hundred cases of cancer of the rectum treated by perineal excision. Br J Surg 14: 110–124
2. Dukes CE (1932) The classification of cancer of the rectum. J Pathol Bacteriol 35: 323–332
3. Astler VB, Coller FA (1954) The prognostic significance of direct extension of carcinoma of colon and rectum. Ann Surg 139: 846–852
4. Dukes CE,Bussey HJR (1958) The spread of rectal cancer and its effect on prognosis. Br J Surg 12: 309–320
5. Pihl E, Hughes ESR, McDermott FT, Milne BJ, Korner JMN, Price AB (1980) Carcinoma of the colon. Cancer specific long-term survival. A series of 615 patients treated by one surgeon. Ann Surg 192: 114–117
6. Pihl E, Hughes ESR, McDermott FT, Milne BJ, Korner JMN, Price AB (1980) Carcinoma of the rectum and rectosigmoid: cancer specific long-term survival. A series of 1061 cases treated by one surgeon. Cancer 45: 2902–2907
7. Newland RC, Chapuis PH, Pheils MT, Macpherson JG (1981) The relationship of survival to staging and grading of colorectal carcinoma: a prospective study of 503 cases. Cancer 47: 1424–1429
8. Blenkinsopp WK, Stewart-Brown S, Blesovsky L, Kearney G, Fielding LP (1981) Histopathology reporting in large bowel cancer. J Clin Pathol 34: 509–513
9. Davis NC, Newland RC (1983) Terminology and classification of colorectal adenocarcinoma: the Australian clinico-pathological staging system. Aust NZ J Surg 53: 211–221
10. Brandao O, Sobrinho-Simoes MA, Serrao D, Moutinho-Ribeiro M, Azevedo C (1985) Prognosis in colorectal carcinoma. A reassessment of the pathologist's role. Pathol Res Pract 180: 506–510
11. Chapuis PH, Dent OF, Fisher R, Newland RC, Pheils MT, Smyth E, Colquhoun K (1985) A multivariate analysis of clinical and pathological variables in prognosis after resection of large bowel cancer. Br J Surg 72: 698–702

12. Fielding LP, Phillips RKS, Fry JS, Hittinger R (1986) Prediction of outcome after curative resection for large bowel cancer. Lancet ii: 904–907
13. Newland RC, Chapuis PH, Smyth EJ (1987) The prognostic value of substaging colorectal carcinoma. A prospective study of 1117 cases with standardized pathology. Cancer 60: 852–857
14. Turnbull RB, Kyle K, Watson FR, Spratt J (1967) Cancer of the colon: the influence of the no-touch isolation technic on survival rates. Ann Surg 166: 420–427
15. Jass JR, Atkin WS, Cuzik J, Bussey HJR, Morson BC, Northover JMA, Todd IP (1986) The grading of rectal cancer: historical perspectives and a multivariate analysis of 447 cases. Histopathology 10: 437–459
16. Jass JR, Love SB, Northover JMA (1987) A new prognostic classification of rectal cancer. Lancet i: 1303–1306
17. Shepherd NA, Saraga EP, Loves SB, Jass JR (1989) Prognostic factors in colonic cancer. Histopathology 14: 613–620
18. Cox D (1972) Regression models and life tables (with discussion). J R Stat Soc [B] 34: 187–220
19. Oota K, Sobin LH (1976) Histological classification of gastric and oesophageal tumours. WHO, Geneva.
20. Ming SC (1977) Gastric carcinoma. A pathobiological classification. Cancer 39: 2475–2485
21. Talbot IC, Ritchie S, Leighton M, Hughes AO, Bussey HJR, Morson BC (1981) Invasion of veins by carcinoma of rectum: method of detection, histological features and significance. Histopathology 5: 141–163

Delay in the Diagnosis and Treatment of Colorectal Cancer

A.R. Dixon and J. Thornton Holmes

Introduction

With over 38 000 cases registered and over 17 000 deaths each year, colorectal cancer has become the second most common malignancy in the United Kingdom [1]. The prognosis of colorectal cancer is primarily determined by the extent of tumour spread at the time of diagnosis [2] and for the last two decades it has remained unchanged, probably due to tumours continuing to present at an advanced stage [3, 4].

During the last decade various developments in diagnostic techniques have taken place, double contrast barium enemas and colonoscopy have become routine examinations. However, despite their availability it has been estimated that some 800 patients die annually in the United Kingdom from the complications of unsuspected colorectal carcinomas, 55% having been thought suitable for a potentially curative resection [5].

In 1968 only 30% of patients with colonic tumours presented to surgeons within 3 months of developing symptoms, 25% of patients with rectal tumours had been symptomatic for over a year [6]. These figures remained unchanged in the decade that followed [7], with delays attributable to both the patient and family doctor alike.

This study was undertaken to assess the accuracy of referral for patients with colorectal carcinomas and to estimate the delay in diagnosis over the last decade. Special emphasis was placed on those patients having malignancies within the ascending colon, distal sigmoid, or rectum.

Patients and Methods

The case notes and medical practitioner referral letters for all 376 consecutive patients with colonic carcinomas electively treated by right hemicolectomy, anterior resection, or abdominoperineal excision of rectum between January 1978 and January 1988, on a single surgical firm at the Peterborough District Hospital were reviewed by the authors. Data collected included: general practitioner's diagnosis; patients symptoms and duration; physical signs; investigations requested; and the time interval to surgery.

Results

Three hundred and seventy-six patients had been referred by 151 general practitioners. A total of 202 rectal tumours were suitable for an anterior resection whilst 85 required an abdominoperineal approach; a right hemicolectomy was performed in the remaining 89 patients. The median age at presentation was 67 years (range 31–91). The mean time interval between development of symptoms and out-patient assessment was 16 weeks for tumours sited in the rectum or distal sigmoid (range 4 days–2 years) and 27 weeks for right-sided carcinomas (range 2–28 months). Surgery was performed on the next available list with a median interval of 20 days (range 3–27 days).

General practitioner-requested barium enemas had been performed in 20 patients; all proved positive. Fourteen patients (8%) experienced a delay in treatment as a consequence of inconclusive barium examinations requested by the surgeons. Rigid sigmoidoscopy was diagnostic in 150 patients.

Rectal and Distal Sigmoid Carcinomas

The presenting symptoms of the 287 patients with rectal and distal sigmoid carcinomas comprised the classic triad: alteration in bowel habit (74%); rectal bleeding (59%) and abdominal pain. Other reported symptoms included perineal discomfort or swelling (14%), weight loss (12%), symptomatic anaemia (4%), abdominal swelling (2%), and disturbed micturition in a further four patients.

Of the 287 patients, 202 had tumours suitable for a sphincter-saving anterior resection and of these 143 (71%) were seen within 2 weeks of receipt of a referral letter that either stated or suggested that the diagnosis was one of cancer. In the remaining patients the general practitioners had attributed symptoms to either: diverticulosis (14%); haemorrhoids (6%); or the irritable bowel syndrome (4%). Eleven patients were referred without commitment to a possible diagnosis. Rectal examination revealed 136 carcinomas, 47% of which had been noted in the general practitioners referral letter. Twelve patients with easily palpable tumours had been referred without a prior rectal examination.

Eighty-five patients required an abdominoperineal excision of rectum with an end colostomy. Analysis of this group's referral letters revealed that 70% had been referred with the correct diagnosis; all stating that a carcinoma was palpable. In spite of having had an apparently normal rectal examination, a further 11 patients were referred for urgent investigation of a possible malignancy. Fifteen patients (17%) in whom rectal examination had been omitted had letters requesting treatment of haemorrhoids; unfortunately these patients were seen routinely, leading to a median delay in diagnosis of 9 weeks.

Right-Sided Colonic Carcinomas

General practitioner referral letters indicted a diagnosis of malignancy in 87% of the 89 patients treated by a right hemicolectomy; 68 referrals had suggested that the carcinoma was sited in the caecum. The mean duration of symptoms up to out-patient assessment was 27 weeks (2–28 months). This delay in presentation was reflected in the symptoms described: symptomatic anaemia (52%); abdominal pain (50%); abdominal mass (40%) and weight loss (14%).

Discussion

The average delay from the onset of symptoms until treatment was reported in 1979 to be 7.5 months, rising to 9 months for patients with rectal malignancies [7]. As a result of this delay 19%–42% of patients will require emergency surgery [4, 7, 8], 76% of these having already consulted their doctor about symptoms on one or more occasions [7]. However, once symptoms have occurred a delay in diagnosis does not necessarily have a detrimental effect upon survival [6, 7] unless emergency surgery becomes mandatory. Emergency surgery is associated with a hospital mortality of 24%, as compared to the 3.6% of elective procedure [9]. Avoidance of emergency surgery may thus improve both morbidity and mortality, particularly in the elderly. Earlier diagnosis may place more patients in the elective group.

Holliday and Hardcastle [7] attributed delays in diagnosis to patients not knowing the importance of bowel symptoms and a failure of their medical practitioner to both recognise the symptoms of colorectal carcinoma and to adequately examine them; 22% of patients with rectal cancer had no rectal examination prior to hospital referral. When medical practitioners were questioned about factors that might cause a delay in referring patients [10], 40% said that a reluctance to refer for unpleasant investigations was a factor as was the age of the patient, particularly if over 75 or under 40 years of age.

This study reports a mean delay of 19 weeks from the onset of symptoms to surgical treatment for rectal and distal sigmoid carcinomas and 29 weeks for carcinomas situated in the ascending colon, a considerable improvement on the 38 and 31 weeks respectively reported in 1979 [7]. This improvement may well be due to an increased recognition by general practitioners of the symptoms that suggest colorectal cancer; 202 patients (70%) with rectal/distal sigmoid tumours and 87% of those with right-sided colonic cancer were referred urgently with the correct diagnosis. This apparently improved accuracy in diagnosing right-sided as compared with rectal malignancies was at the expense of a more prolonged period of symptoms, possibly representing a lack of patient awareness as to the importance of their more general ill health.

Of the lesions palpated per rectum by the surgeons, 56% had been detected by the general practitioner, including 70% of the low rectal tumours. However, 12% of patients with easily palpable carcinomas had been referred with letters attributing their symptoms to "piles"; in each case a rectal examination had been omitted. Unfortunately these patients were seen on a routine basis, and as a result their treatment was delayed.

Although we have shown an improvement in referrals over this 10-year period compared with 1979 [7] the performance of a rectal examination in each patient would have improved matters further.

References

1. Office of Population and Surveys (1981) Cancer Research Campaign Cancer Statistics. Incidence, Survival and Mortality in England and Wales. Studies on Medical and Population Subjects N° 43. HMSO, London, viii, xii, pp 22–29
2. Chapuis PH, Dent OF, Fisher R, Newland RC, Pheils MT, Smyth E, Colquhoun K (1985) A multivariate analysis of clinical and pathological variables in prognosis after resection of large bowel cancer. Br J Surg 72: 698–702
3. Stower MJ, Hardcastle JD (1985) The results of 1115 patients with colorectal cancer treated over an 8-year period in a single hospital. Eur J Surg Oncol 11: 119–123
4. Umpleby HC, Bristol JB, Rainey JB, Williamson RCN (1984) Survival of 727 patients with single carcinomas of the large bowel. Dis Colon Rectum 27: 803–810
5. Armstrong CP, Whitelaw SJ (1989) Death from unsuspected colorectal cancer. Ann R Coll Surg Engl 71: 20–22
6. Keddie N, Hargreaves A (1968) Symptoms of carcinoma of the colon and rectum. Lancet ii: 749–750
7. Holliday HW, Hardcastle JD (1979) Delay in diagnosis and treatment of symptomatic colorectal cancer. Lancet i: 309–311
8. Umpleby HC, Williamson RCN (1984) Survival in acute obstructing colorectal carcinoma. Dis Colon Rectum 27: 299–304
9. Till AS (1977) The results of treatment in district general hospitals. Top Gastroenterol 3: 77–89
10. Nichols S (1986) General practitioners' awareness of colorectal cancer. Br Med J 292: 308–310

Potentiation of the Antiproliferative Effect of 5′-Deoxy-5-Fluorouridine by Interferon-Alpha 2a

H. Tevaearai, P. Laurent, L. Suardet, J. Eliason, J.-C. Givel, and N. Odartchenko

Introduction

Fluoropyrimidines are commonly used in clinical oncology, but their strong dose-dependent toxicity limits therapeutic application. The synthetic derivative 5′-deoxy-5-fluorouridine (5′-dFUrd) [1] has raised marked interest due to a higher therapeutic index as compared with 5-fluorouracil (5-FUra) or other related compounds [2–4]. It is also a less potent leukopenia inducer [2, 5] and is not as strongly immunosuppressive as other fluoropyrimidines [6, 7]. The biological activity of this pro-drug is dependent upon its enzymatic cleavage to 5-FUra by a pyrimidine phosphorylase [8–10] which is found in much higher levels in human and animal tumours than in normal tissues, except in the intestinal tract [3, 4, 10–12].

Recently, the combination of interferon-α (IFN-α) plus 5-FUra has been shown to give objective responses in 13 of 17 previously untreated patients with advanced colorectal carcinoma [13, 14]. This prompted us to analyse the in vitro effects of IFN-α on the cytotoxicity of 5-FUra and of the pro-drug 5′-dFUrd with human colon carcinoma cell lines. Potentiation of the effect of 5-FUra by IFN-α was seen in only one out of six cell lines, but the combination of IFN-α with the pro-drug 5′-dFUrd was synergistic in four cell lines. We have been able to correlate this synergism with 5′-dFUrd with the induction of higher levels of pyrimidine phosphorylase activity by IFN-α.

Materials and Methods

Cell Lines

Six colon cell lines derived from primary human tumours (WiDr, HT-29, SW-480. LISP-1, Co-115 and 513) were cultured in a 1:1 mixture of enriched Dulbecoo's modified Eagle's medium (EMED) and modified Ham's F-12 nutrient mixture (FMED) supplemented with 10% fetal calf serum [15].

Drugs

Recombinant human IFN-α 2A (Roferon A), 5-FUra and 5′-dFUrd were provided by Hoffman-La Roche, Basel, Switzerland. IFN-α was tested in three arbitrarily defined concentrations (100; 1000; 10000 IU/ml).

Methodology

Experiments were done in triplicate, using a liquid proliferation assay in microtiter plates (96 wells). One thousand cells were plated at day 0; drugs or drug combinations were added on day 3 and relative cell numbers were determined after five more days by the (4,5-dimethylthiazol-2-yl)-2,5-diphenyltetrazolium bromide (MTT) spectrophotometric assay. Plates were incubated at 37°C in a 95% humidified incubator with 5% CO_2. Titration curves were obtained for each cell line, in order to correlate measured optical density with absolute cell number. The least-square regression lines for log(survival) vs drug combination were used to calculate the IC_{50}. Results obtained with drug combinations were corrected for the inhibitory effect of IFN-α alone.

Pyrimidine Phosphorylase Activity

This was measured by the method of Choong et al. [16], which is based on differences in ultraviolet (UV) absorption spectra of 5′-dFUrd and 5-FUra, and which focuses on the ability of pyrimidine phosphorylase to convert the substrate 5′d-FUrd to 5-FUra.

Results and Discussion

The biological activity of the pro-drug 5′-dFUrd depends upon its intracellular enzymatic cleavage by pyrimidine phosphorylase to form 5-FUra. In our study, sensitivity to 5-FUra was not significantly different between the cell lines tested, but growth inhibitory effect of the pro-drug 5′-dFUrd varied widely from one cell line to the other (Tables 1 and 2). Activity of pyrimidine phosphorylase was therefore analysed (Table 3) by focusing on its ability to convert the substrate 5′-dFUrd to 5-FUra, and appeared to be strictly correlated to the effect of the pro-drug 5′-dFUrd. The activity of pyrimidine phosphorylase is thus determinant for activity of 5′-dFUrd.

IFN-α has been shown to increase the cytotoxic effects of 5-FUra in vitro [17–22] and in vivo in mice [23] and in humans [13, 14, 24]. We also

Table 1. Effect of IFN-α on inhibitory activity (IC_{50}) of 5-FUra[a] against human colorectal cancer cell lines[b]

Cell line	0 IU/ml	100 IU/ml	1000 IU/ml	10 000 IU/ml
WiDr	1.25 ± 0.46	1.12 ± 0.51	1.32 ± 0.43	1.24 ± 0.46
HT-29	0.91 ± 0.36	0.79 ± 0.37	0.97 ± 0.44	0.88 ± 0.36
513	0.64 ± 0.29	0.62 ± 0.28	0.66 ± 0.26	0.66 ± 0.25
Co-115	1.16 ± 0.35	1.14 ± 0.33	0.94 ± 0.40	1.26 ± 0.35
LISP-1	0.79 ± 0.31	0.86 ± 0.30	0.84 ± 0.39	0.83 ± 0.37
SW-480	0.75 ± 0.31	0.52 ± 0.24	0.40 ± 0.24	0.35 ± 0.23

[a] Expressed in μg/ml
[b] Results are the mean of at least three different experiences

Table 2. Effect of IFN-α on inhibitory activity (IC_{50}) of 5′-dFUrd[a] against human colorectal cancer cell lines[b]

Cell line	0 IU/ml	100 IU/ml	1000 IU/ml	10 000 IU/ml
WiDr	93.4 ± 36.7	54.7 ± 22.1	45.7 ± 20.1	39.4 ± 19.5
HT-29	93.4 ± 39.2	77.2 ± 41.5	77.8 ± 30.8	58.9 ± 36.1
513	21.2 ± 8.5	15.3 ± 8.6	14.3 ± 6.4	12.8 ± 5.6
Co-115	2.3 ± 0.4	1.8 ± 0.6	1.5 ± 0.4	1.1 ± 0.3
LISP-1	11.3 ± 2.3	12.0 ± 3.3	11.6 ± 3.2	10.7 ± 3.6
SW-480	56.9 ± 33.6	53.8 ± 29.7	47.1 ± 25.3	37.4 ± 24.8

[a] Expressed in μg/ml
[b] Results are the mean of at least three different experiences

Table 3. Effect of IFN-α on pyrimidine phosphorylase activity[a,b]

Cell line	0 IU/ml	100 IU/ml	1000 IU/ml	10 000 IU/ml
WiDr	0.84 ± 0.13	1.05 ± 0.29	1.60 ± 0.24	1.84 ± 0.09
HT-29	0.71 ± 0.03	1.03 ± 0.09	1.07 ± 0.10	1.91 ± 0.32
513	1.42 ± 0.16	1.77 ± 0.26	2.31 ± 0.39	3.09 ± 0.39
Co-115	2.46 ± 0.17	3.04 ± 0.53	4.41 ± 0.32	5.98 ± 0.23
LISP-1	1.63 ± 0.48	1.84 ± 0.60	1.71 ± 0.55	1.81 ± 0.55
SW-480	0.93 ± 0.15	0.99 ± 0.23	1.01 ± 0.21	1.19 ± 0.15

[a] Expressed in μmol of 5-FUra formed, normalized to grams of proteins and minutes of incubation
[b] Results are the mean of three different experiences

found evidence of synergy between IFN-α and 5-FUra (Table 1), but only in one out of six colorectal tumour cell lines (SW-480). However, in four of the five other lines (WiDr, HT-29, 513 and Co-115), a synergistic effect was seen with the combination of IFN-α and the pro-drug 5′-dFUrd only (Table 2) but not with 5-FUra (Table 1). These differential effects suggest that IFN-α might modulate cleavage of 5′-dFUrd to 5-FUra by enhancing the activity of pyrimidine phosphorylase. We therefore determined this activity in cells previously treated with IFN-α. The results confirm that cell lines showing a synergistic effect between 5′-dFUrd and IFN-α (WiDr, HT-29, 513 and Co-115) exhibit enhanced pyrimidine phosphorylase activity, while no change is noted in one cell line (LISP-1) where no synergy occurred. Stimulation of pyrimidine phosphorylase activity thus appears to be one major mechanism through which IFN-α potentiates the effect of 5′-dFUrd.

Although synergy between IFN-α and 5-FUra was confirmed in one cell line, our results suggest that direct effect of IFN-α on tumour cells is more evident with the pro-drug 5′-dFUrd. Activity of pyrimidine phosphorylase, which is determinant for activity of 5′-dFUrd, can be stimulated by IFN-α in converting 5′-dFUrd to 5-FUra, leading to improved efficacy of the pro-drug. With regard to the encouraging clinical results of Wadler et al. [13, 14], combined treatment using this pro-drug together with IFN-α might further improve the therapeutic index, particularly in resistant tumours such as those of the gastrointestinal tract.

References

1. Cook AF, Holman MJ, Kramer MJ, Trown PW (1979) Fluorinated pyrimidine nucleosides. III. Synthesis and antitumor activity of a series of 5′-deoxy-5-fluoropyrimidine nucleosides. J Med Chem 22: 1330–1335
2. Bollag W, Hartmann HR (1980) Tumor inhibitory effects of a new fluorouracil derivative: 5′-deoxy-5-fluorouridine. Eur J Cancer 16: 427–432
3. Armstrong RD, Diasio RB (1981) Selective activation of 5′-deoxy-5-fluorouridine by tumor cells as a basis for an improved therapeutic index. Cancer Res 41: 4891–4894
4. Armstrong RD, Cadman E (1983) 5′-deoxy-5-fluorouridine selective toxicity for human tumor cells compared to human bone marrow. Cancer Res 43: 2525–2528
5. Kramer MJ, Trown PW, Cleeland R, Cook AF, Grunberg E (1979) 5′-deoxy-5-fluorouridine, a new orally active antitumor agent. Comparative activity with 5-fluorouracil, 2′-deoxy-5-fluorouridine and ftorafur against transplantable tumors in mice and rats. Proc Am Assoc Cancer Res 20: 79
6. Connolly KM, Diasio RB, Armstrong RD, Kaplan AM (1983) Decreased immunosuppression associated with antitumor activity of 5-deoxy-5-fluorouridine compared to 5-fluorouracil and 5-fluorouridine. Cancer Res 43: 2529–2535
7. Ohta Y, Sueki K, Kitta K, Takemoto K, Ishitsuka H, Yagi Y (1980) Comparative studies on the immunosuppressive effect among 5′-deoxy-5-fluorouridine, ftorafur, and 5-fluorouracil. Jpn J Cancer Res 71: 190–196
8. Armstrong RD, Diasio RB (1980) Metabolism and biological activity of 5′-deoxy-5-fluorouridine, a novel fluoropyrimidine. Cancer Res 40: 3333–3338

9. Ishitsuka H, Miwa M, Takemoto K, Fukuoka K, Itoga A, Maruyama HB (1980) Role of uridine phosphorylase for antitumor activity of 5′-deoxy-5-fluorouridine. Jpn J Cancer Res 71: 112–123
10. Kono A, Hara Y, Sugata S, Karube Y, Matsushima Y, Ishitsuka H (1983) Activation of 5′-deoxy-5-fluorouridine by thymidine phosphorylase in human tumors. Chem Pharm Bull (Tokyo) 31: 175–178
11. Suzuki S, Hongu Y, Fukazawa H, Ichihara S, Shimizu H (1980) Tissue distribution of 5′-deoxy-5-fluorouridine and derived 5-fluorouracil in tumor-bearing mice and rats. Jpn J Cancer Res 71: 238–245
12. Choong YS, Lee SP, Alley PA (1988) Comparison of the pyrimidine nucleoside phosphorylase activity in human tumors and normal tissues. Exp Pathol 33: 23–25
13. Wadler S, Schwartz EL, Goldman M, Lyver A, Rader M, Zimmerman M, Itri L, Weinberg V, Wiernik PH (1989) Fluorouracil and recombinant alpha-2a-interferon: an active regimen against advanced colorectal carcinoma. J Clin Oncol 7: 1769–1775
14. Wadler S, Wiernik PH (1990) Clinical update on the role of fluorouracil and recombinant interferon alpha-2a in the treatment of colorectal carcinoma. Semin Oncol 17: 16–21
15. Eliason JF, Aapro MS, Decrey D, Brink-Petersen M (1985) Non-linearity of colony formation by human tumor cells from biopsy samples. Br J Cancer 52: 311–318
16. Choong YS, Lee SP (1985) The degradation of 5′-deoxy-5-fluorouridine by pyrimidine nucleoside phosphorylase in normal and cancer tissues. Clin Chim Acta 149: 175–183
17. Namba M, Miyoshi T, Kanamori T, Nobuhara M, Kimoto T, Ogawa S (1982) Combined effects of 5-fluorouracil and interferon on proliferation of human neoplastic cells in culture. Jpn J Cancer Res 73: 819–824
18. Sato M, Yoshida H, Urata M, Yanagawa T, Yura Y, Nitta T, Kobayashi S, Hayashi Y (1984) Effect of 5-fluorouracil and the combination of 5-fluorouracil and human leukocyte interferon on human salivary gland adenocarcinoma cell line in culture. Int J Oral Surg 13: 35–44
19. Yamamoto S, Tanaka H, Kanamori T, Nobuhara M, Namba M (1983) In vitro studies on potentiation of cytotoxic effects of anticancer drugs by interferon on a human neoplastic cell line (HeLa). Cancer Lett 20: 131–138
20. Miyoshi T, Ogawa S, Kanamori T, Nobuhara M, Namba M (1983) Interferon potentiates cytotoxic effects of 5-fluorouracil on cell proliferation of established human cell lines originating from neoplastic tissues. Cancer Lett 17: 239–247
21. Elias L, Crissman HA (1988) Interferon effects upon the adenocarcinoma 38 and HL-60 cell lines: antiproliferative responses and synergistic interactions with halogenated pyrimidine antimetabolites. Cancer Res 48: 4868–4873
22. Elias L, Sandoval JM (1989) Interferon effects upon fluorouracil metabolism by HL-60 cells. Biochem Biophys Res Commun 163: 867–874
23. Birsic W, d'Oro L, Charoensiri S, Katoh A (1989) The combined effect of interferon and 5-FU on tumor-cell metastasis in the nude mouse. Dis Colon Rectum 32: 340–343
24. de Vecchis L, Nunziata C, Ricci F, Cucchiara G, Picconi A, Bonmassar G, Lagomarsino Caprino M, Bonmassar E (1989) Immunochemotherapy of advanced colorectal cancer with α-interferon and 5-fluorouracil. 1. Toxicological studies. J Chemother 1: 128–135

Lymph Node Metastases in Early Rectal Cancer

S.P.J. Huddy, R. Sexton, E.M. Husband and R.J. Heald

Introduction

Local removal of rectal carcinoma has been recommended as a definitive procedure in the treatment of early rectal cancer [1–3]. However this procedure does not remove local lymph nodes in the mesorectum, thus preventing full staging of the tumour and removing the prospect of cure for those patients with involved nodes.

This study is designed to clarify the incidence of metastatic lymph node spread in early rectal carcinoma and to investigate whether features of the primary tumour can be used to predict which patients will have nodal involvement.

Methods

We have reviewed the histological findings of a consecutive series of 220 rectums removed for cancer in a single hospital. In each case the tumour was removed by either a radical anterior approach involving a wide mesorectal clearance or by an abdomino-perineal operation.

The tumours which were reported as Dukes' stage C were identified and studied to identify those in which the primary tumour had not penetrated through the muscularis propria. The local features of these tumours were then compared to the Dukes' A tumours in the series.

Results

The series comprised 220 cases. There were 85 (39%) Dukes' stage C, 89 (40%) stage B and 46 (21%) stage A tumours. Eight of the 46 stage A tumours were described as being polypoid.

Fifty-six cases were identified where the primary tumour did not penetrate through the muscularis propria. Ten (18%) of these had secondary deposits within local lymph nodes and were thus reported as C tumours.

Table 1. The features of primary rectal tumours locally confined to the bowel wall with or without metastatic node involvement

	Node positive	Node negative	P value
Tumour height (cm)	5.35 (2.9)	7.59 (3.4)	ns
Tumour diameter (cm)	3.05 (1.4)	4.15 (1.6)	$p < .05$
Depth of tumour penetration (cm)			
Mucosa	0	7	ns
Submucosa	1	7	
Muscularis propria	9	32	
Degree of tumour differentiation			
Well	3	21	ns
Moderate	4	19	
Poor	3	6	

Values in parentheses are standard deviation
ns, not significant

The tumour diameter, distance of tumour from the anal margin, depth of tumour penetration and degree of cellular differentiation for the 56 tumours locally confined to the bowel wall are given in Table 1.

Discussion

Local removal of rectal tumours is an attractive proposition. The surgery involved is relatively minor with a correspondingly low morbidity and mortality and may avoid a temporary or permanent stoma. The technique however does not remove mesorectal lymph nodes. The histological examination of these nodes when removed allows staging and an estimate of prognosis. More importantly wide clearance of these nodes "in continuity" with the primary can frequently be curative [4].

When considering a local resection, the risks of incomplete tumour removal must be weighed against the morbidity and mortality of a radical operation. In our series of patients the 5-year survival after curative anterior resection for all patients with C tumours is approximately 60%. The operative mortality for patients under 70 years of age undergoing curative surgery is approximately 1%. Clearly when the involved lymph nodes are left behind surgery cannot be expected to be curative.

Furthermore there is some evidence to suggest that Dukes' C tumours in which the primary does not penetrate through the bowel wall have a better prognosis than C tumours as a whole. Wolmark et al. [5] reported fewer involved nodes (mean 2.5 vs 4) and more patients having only one involved node (47% vs 15%) when the primary was confined to the bowel wall. Copeland et al. [6] reported a 53% 5-year survival for this group as opposed to 20% when the tumour penetrated the wall and as long ago as 1954 Astler and Coller [7] reported a 42.8% and 22.4% 5-year survival respectively.

It is unfortunately not possible at present to accurately predict preoperatively which patients will have nodal metastases. Digital rectal examination has been shown to be an unreliable guide [8]. Computed tomography (CT) scanning is useful in determining local depth of invasion and the presence of distant metastases but is disappointing in its ability to detect tumour in local lymph nodes [9, 10], proving little better than digital examination [8]. Transrectal echosonography may prove to be a more useful investigation for the detection of nodal metastases. Beynon et al. [10] have reported a series of 49 patients with positive nodes with only five false negative investigations. However the procedure relies upon a high degree of expertise and general results are likely to be less satisfactory.

From our study there was no significant difference in the tumour height, the degree of cellular differentiation or depth of penetration between the tumours with and without lymph node metastases. Although the node negative tumours tended to be larger and this difference reached statistical significance, the magnitude of the difference is small and is of little clinical use.

Present methods of investigation do not allow accurate prediction of those patients who have metastases in local lymph nodes. Features of the local tumour may provide a guide but are unreliable in the specific case. When dealing with a lesion which is curable in the majority of cases by adequate surgery, the risks of conservative surgery must be appreciated and taken into account when planning the optimal treatment for each individual patient.

References

1. Mason AY (1976) Role of local surgery in carcinoma of the rectum. Proc R Soc Med 69: 869–872
2. Morson BC, Bussey HJR, Samoorian S (1977) Policy of local excision for early cancer of the colorectum. Gut 18: 1045–1050
3. Horn A, Halvorsen JF, Morild I (1989) Transanal extirpation for early rectal cancer. Dis Colon Rectum 32: 769–772
4. Heald RJ, Ryall RDH (1986) Recurrence and survival after total mesorectal excision for rectal cancer. Lancet i: 1479–1482
5. Wolmark N, Fisher ER, Wieland S, Fisher B (1984) The relationship of depth of penetration and tumor size to the number of positive nodes in Dukes C colorectal cancer. Cancer 53: 2707–2712
6. Copeland EM, Miller LD, Jones RS (1968) Prognostic factors in carcinoma of the colon and rectum. Am J Surg 116: 875–881
7. Astler VB, Coller FA (1954) Prognostic significance of direct extension of carcinoma of colon and rectum. Ann Surg 139: 846–852
8. Nicholls RJ, York Mason A, Morson BC, Dixon AK, Kelsey Fry I (1982) The clinical staging of rectal cancer. Br J Surg 69: 404–409
9. Thoeni RF (1989) CT evaluation of carcinomas of the colon and rectum. Radiol Clin North Am 27: 731–741
10. Beynon J, Mortensen NJ McC, Foy DMA, Channer JL, Rigby H, Virjee J (1989) Preoperative assessment of mesorectal lymph node involvement in rectal cancer. Br J Surg 76: 276–279

Modification of DNA Ploidy in Rectal Cancer Following Pre-Operative Radiotherapy

M.J.C. Matter, S. Rowley and G.D. Oates

Introduction

Recent studies on colorectal cancer [1–6] and on rectal cancer alone [7–10] using flow cytometry analysis have demonstrated the prognostic role of DNA stemline assessment. Selected patients who underwent a curative resection for a DNA aneuploid tumour had a higher local recurrence rate and a lower survival rate. DNA content of pre-operative biopsies may reflect the content of the resected primary [11] and thus afford an additional factor in pre-operative staging, as proposed by Williams et al. [12].

Tumour heterogeneity is a well-known problem in colorectal cancer. Multiple DNA stemlines are encountered in about a third of the DNA aneuploid cases [11, 13–16]. According to Quirke's and Williams' studies, superficial sampling does not differ consistently from a deep one [12, 15].

A recent review on adjuvant radiotherapy by Twomey et al. in 1989 showed that a reduction of up to 40% in local recurrence rate could be achieved [17]. Patients with a bad prognosis, based partly on DNA ploidy status, may be selected for such adjuvant therapy.

Few studies have compared pre-operative biopsies with resected tumours from a DNA ploidy point of view. We have reviewed and compared pre-operative samples with those from irradiated tumours to observe if DNA ploidy could be a response marker. With the help of the literature we have tried to answer two questions: can flow cytometry reflect the response to radiotherapy and is ploidy of the irradiated tumour still representative of its biology?

Patients, Materials and Methods

We have reviewed retrospectively 31 patients (16 men and 15 women, mean age 63.3 years), operated on for primary rectal adenocarcinoma. All but two had a pre-operative biopsy showing an invasive adenocarcinoma; the other two showed severe dysplasia. Twenty-one had an anterior restorative resection and ten an abdomino-perineal resection. Twenty-three patients had pre-operative radiotherapy (40–50 Gy), mainly under the protocol of the Medical Research Council 2 (MRC 2) trial for locally advanced rectal tumours. The radiotherapy group had surgery with a 4- to 6-weeks delay. Eight patients were randomized into a surgery only group, and their specimens were analysed to demonstrate tumour heterogeneity between pre-operative biopsies and resected primaries.

Slides of all available paraffin-embedded blocks have been reviewed to select sections with at least 10%–20% of tumour cells. The 182 samples obtained included pre-operative biopsies, at least two samples of the resected primaries, metastatic lymph nodes, liver metastases and normal lymph nodes or large bowel (proximal resected margin) as diploid controls.

Preparation of the cell suspension roughly followed the method described by Hedley et al. [18]. Two to four slices 30–40 µm thick were prepared from the selected blocks. The sections were dewaxed in two changes of xylene (10–15 min each), rehydrated in decreasing concentrations of ethanol (100%, 95%, 70% and 50%; 10 min each), and then rinsed twice in distilled water for 10 min each time. The cells were obtained following incubation in 0.5% pepsin in 0.9% NaCl for 30 min in a 37°C water bath. The solutions were centrifuged twice. The cells were then filtered through a 35-µm nylon mesh, centrifuged again and resuspended in 1 ml of propidium iodide for at least 30 min.

Cellular DNA content was measured with a flow cytometer (FACS IV, Becton-Dickinson, Sunnyvale, California, USA) on 20 000–30 000 cells, and analysed with the incorporated computer. In given coefficient of variation greater than 10 the sample was repeated. On each histogram the first peak was taken to represent a normal diploid population. Any other containing at least 10% of the total number of nuclei was considered a DNA aneuploid peak. The DNA index (DI) was calculated as the ratio of the aneuploid G_0/G_1 fluorescence channel peak to the first diploid G_0/G_1 fluorescence channel peak. The chi-squared test was used for tables analysis.

Results

There were 0, 9, 11 and 11 Dukes' stage A, B, C and D adenocarcinomas, respectively. Eight biopsies (26%) were DNA aneuploid and 23 (74%) diploid. The mean (SD) coefficient of variation was 8.2% (1.2). A mean of 2.4 blocks were analysed from each primary. The mean (SD) coefficient of variation was 8.4% (1.4). Overall 11 primaries (35%) were DNA aneuploid and 20 (65%) diploid. Four out of eight tumours (50%) were DNA aneuploid in the surgery only group, and 7 out of 23 (30%) in the radiotherapy group. The difference is however not significant (Table 1).

We then compared the ploidy results in the two treatment groups. The tumours of eight patients having no pre-operative radiotherapy were studied

Table 1. Tumour DNA ploidy and adjuvant radiotherapy[a]

	DNA diploid		DNA aneuploid	
	n	%	*n*	%
Radiotherapy group (n = 23)	16	70	7	30
Surgery only group (n = 8)	4	50	4	50

[a] Analysis using $\chi^2 = 0.99$; differences were not significant between the two groups

Table 2. DNA ploidy of preoperative biopsies and resected primaries in the surgery only group of eight patients

Biopsy		Primary	
DNA ploidy	*n*	DNA ploidy	*n*
DNA aneuploid	1	DNA aneuploid	1
DNA diploid	7	DNA aneuploid	3[a]
		DNA diploid	4

[a] Two lesions with demonstrated heterogeneity

Table 3. DNA ploidy of preoperative biopsies and resected primaries in the radiotherapy group of 23 patients

Biopsy		Primary	
DNA ploidy	*n*	DNA ploidy	*n*
DNA aneuploid	7	DNA aneuploid	5[a]
		DNA diploid	2
DNA diploid	16	DNA aneuploid	2[b]
		DNA diploid	14

[a] Four primaries with demonstrated heterogeneity
[b] One primary with demonstrated heterogeneity

as controls. One biopsy was DNA aneuploid and seven DNA diploid; but after resection, three lesions were DNA aneuploid, two with demonstrated DNA stemline heterogeneity (Table 2).

Among 23 patients receiving pre-operative radiotherapy, 16 had a diploid biopsy, but two of these had a DNA aneuploid primary, one with demonstrated heterogeneity. In seven patients with a DNA aneuploid biopsy, five showed no change, four of them with demonstrated heterogeneity. Only two had a DNA diploid resected tumour (Table 3).

Our small series, comprising 35 palliative resections, did not allow for a survival analysis.

In the surgery only group (Table 2) we may conclude that three out of eight samples were wrongly assessed pre-operatively, and that a more usual 50% (4/8) DNA aneuploid proportion would be the correct allocation. Applying this figure to the radiotherapy group would allocate six further samples to the DNA aneuploid group of biopsies. The two possible changes of ploidy may therefore be an underestimate of the actual state of affairs (Table 3).

Discussion

According to Remvikos et al. [19] there is a good correlation between cytogenetic and flow cytometry analysis for DNA content in colorectal cancer. Numerous reports have applied and developed Hedley's procedure for paraffin-embedded blocks. Their results are well reproducible and similar to those obtained with fresh tumour cells [1, 20].

Tumour heterogeneity may be illustrated by the demonstration of DNA multiple stemlines. About 60% of colorectal adenocarcinomas are DNA aneuploid, one third of these being DNA heterogenous [13, 14, 16]. Quirke et al. [15] estimated that 72% of malignancies were correctly assessed with a unique sample, which is more than we have found. The prognostic role of DNA stemline heterogeneity remains to be determined [2, 8].

Although two biopsies showed severe dysplasia only, DNA aneuploidy and ploidy heterogeneity have been described in such lesions [21].

The lower proportion of DNA aneuploid cancer in the radiotherapy group (Table 1) confirms the significant data obtained by Jones et al. in a similar study (37% in the radiotherapy group versus 62% in the surgery only group, $p < 0.01$). He observed a significant increased survival rate for patients with a DNA diploid tumour, but only in the surgery only group. A DNA aneuploid primary in the radiotherapy group was a significant predictor for local recurrence [22].

At least two patients with a DNA aneuploid biopsy had a DNA diploid primary following radiotherapy, which may indicate a biological response. A recent review of the literature showed that efficacy of radiotherapy has only been assessed by such an analysis in gynaecological tumours [23, 24].

Bliven et al. proved in a biological study that cellular heterogeneity implicates multiple clone radiosensitivity [25]. However, there seems to be no direct relationship between radiosensitivity and DNA content [26].

Provided good biopsy sampling is obtained, DNA analysis may help in assessing the effect of pre-operative radiotherapy.

References

1. Armitage NC, Robins RA, Evans DF, Turner DR, Baldwin RW, Hartcastle JD (1985) The influence of tumour cell DNA abnormalities on survival in colorectal cancer. Br J Surg 72: 828–830
2. Bauer KD, Lincoln ST, Vera-Roman JM, Wallemark CB, Chmiel JS, Madurski ML, Murad T, Scarpelli DG (1987) Prognostic implications of proliferative activity and DNA aneuploidy in colonic adenocarcinomas. Lab Invest 57: 329–335
3. Scott NA, Wieand HS, Moertel CG, Cha SS, Beart RW, Lieber MM (1987) Colorectal cancer. Dukes' stage, tumor site, preoperative plasma CEA level, and patient prognosis related to tumor DNA ploidy pattern. Arch Surg 122: 1375–1379
4. Jones DJ, Moore M, Schofield PF (1988) Prognostic significance of DNA ploidy in colorectal cancer: a prospective flow cytometric study. Br J Surg 75: 28–33
5. Wiggers T, Arends JW, Schutte B, Volovics L, Bosman FT (1988) A multivariate analysis of pathologic prognostic indicators in large bowel cancer. Cancer 61: 368–395
6. Kokal WA, Gardine RL, Sheibani K, Morris PL, Prager E, Zak IW, Terz JJ (1989) Tumor DNA content in resectable, primary colorectal carcinoma. Ann Surg 209: 188–193
7. Scott NA, Rainwater LM, Wieand HS, Weiland LH, Pemberton JH, Beart RW, Lieber MM (1987) The relative prognostic value of flow cytometric DNA analysis and conventional clinicopathologic criteria in patients with operable rectal carcinoma. Dis Colon Rectum 30: 513–520
8. Quirke P, Dixon MF, Clayden AD, Durdey P, Dyson JE, Williams NS, Bird CC (1987) Prognostic significance of DNA aneuploidy and cell proliferation in rectal adenocarcinomas. J Pathol 151: 285–291
9. Goh HS, Jass JR, Atkin WS, Cuzick J, Northover JM (1987) Value of flow cytometric determination of ploidy as a guide to prognosis in operable rectal cancer: a multivariate analysis. Int J Colorectal Dis 2: 17–21
10. Fisher ER, Siderits RH, Sass R, Fisher B (1989) Value of assessment of ploidy in rectal cancers. Arch Pathol Lab Med 113: 525–528
11. Scott NA, Grande JP, Weiland LH, Pemberton JH, Beart RW, Lieber MM (1987) Flow cytometric DNA patterns from colorectal cancers – how reproducible are they? Mayo Clin Proc 62: 331–337
12. Williams NS, Durdey P, Quirke P, Robinson PJ, Dyson JE, Dixon MF, Bird CC (1985) Pre-operative staging of rectal neoplasm and its impact on clinical management. Br J Surg 72: 868–874
13. Petersen SE, Lorentzen M, Bichel P (1980) A mosaic subpopulation structure of human colorectal carcinomas demonstrated by flow cytometry. In: Laerum OD et al. (eds) Flow cytometry IV. Universitetsforlaget, Bergen, pp 412–416
14. Tribukait B, Hammarberg C, Rubio C (1983) Ploidy and proliferation patterns in colorectal adenocarcinomas related to Dukes' classification and to histopathological differentiation. A flow-cytometric DNA study. Acta Pathol Microbiol Immunol Scand 91: 89–95
15. Quirke P, Dyson JE, Dixon MF, Bird CC, Joslin CA (1985) Heterogeneity of colorectal adenocarcinomas evaluated by flow cytometry and histopathology. Br J Cancer 51: 99–106
16. Hiddemann W, von Bassewitz DB, Kleinemeier HJ, Schulte-Brochterbeck E, Hauss J, Lingemann B, Büchner T, Grundmann E (1986) DNA stemline heterogeneity in colorectal cancer. Cancer 58: 258–263
17. Twomey P, Burchell M, Strawn D, Guernsey J (1989) Local control in rectal cancer. Arch Surg 124: 1174–1179
18. Hedley DW, Friedlander ML, Taylor IW, Rugg CA, Musgrove EA (1983) Method for analysis of cellular DNA content of paraffin-embedded pathological material using flow cytometry. J Histochem Cytochem 31: 1333–1335

19. Remvikos Y, Muleris M, Vielh P, Salmon RJ, Dutrillaux B (1988) DNA content and genetic evolution of human colorectal adenocarcinoma. A study by flow cytometry and cytogenetic analysis. Int J Cancer 42: 539–543
20. Kute TE, Gregory B, Galleshaw J, Hopkins M, Buss D, Case D (1988) How reproducible are flow cytometry data from paraffin-embedded blocks? Cytometry 9: 494–498
21. Hamada S, Itoh R, Fujita S (1988) DNA distribution pattern of the so-called severe dysplasias and small carcinomas of the colon and rectum and its possible significance in the tumor progression. Cancer 61: 1555–1562
22. Jones DJ, Zaloudik J, James RD, Haboubi N, Moore M, Schofield PF (1989) Predicting local recurrence of carcinoma of the rectum after preoperative radiotherapy and surgery. Br J Surg 76: 1172–1175
23. Izutsu T, Kagabu T, Nishiya I, Wied GL (1988) Retrospective DNA analysis by rapid high resolution cytometry in cases with cervical cancer before and after radiotherapy. Nippon Sanka Fujinka Gakkai Zasshi 40: 909–914
24. Izutsu T, Kagabu T, Nishiya I, Wied GL (1988) DNA analysis cervical and vaginal cancer cells during radiotherapy by rapid high-resolution cytometry. Nippon Sanka Fujinka Gakkai Zasshi 40: 621–626
25. Bliven SF, Schneiderman TE, Leith JT (1987) Cell cycle responses of heterogeneous human colon adenocarcinoma subpopulations to X-irradiation. Cell Tissue Kinet 20: 473–483
26. Schwartz JL, Rotmensch J, Giovanazzi S, Cohen MB, Weichselbaum RR (1988) Faster repair of DNA double-strand breaks in radioresistant human tumor cells. Int J Radiat Oncol Biol Phys 15: 907–912

Bromodeoxyuridine Labelling: A Novel Biomarker of Colon Cancer Risk

R.G. WILSON

Introduction

Autoradiography following ^{3}H-Thymidine (^{3}H-T) incorporation into mucosal fragments in vitro has been widely employed in the study of cell proliferation in subjects at increased risk for colonic neoplasia [1]. Using this technique significant differences in the labelling index (LI) and distribution of proliferative cells within large-bowel crypts have been described in hereditary non-polyposis colon cancer [2], familial polyposis [3] and in the presence of sporadic polyps or carcinoma [4]. In vitro ^{3}H-T labelling has therefore been proposed as a potential method for identification of high risk subjects [4], and has also been used as an "intermediate biomarker" of colon cancer risk in assessing the short-term effects of dietary intervention in man [5]. However it is an exacting technique which requires the use of radioactive isotopes and significant delays (often several weeks) whilst autoradiographs are developed.

The development of a monoclonal antibody against the thymidine analogue, bromodeoxyuridine (Brdu), permits the rapid identification of S-phase cells (and thus the LI) by immunohistochemical techniques [6]. We have assessed its use for in vitro labelling of human colorectal mucosa.

The purpose of the present study was twofold, firstly to compare the LI and pattern of labelling throughout the large-bowel mucosa in normal controls and patients with adenomas and secondly to establish the accuracy of a simple technique for comparison of the proliferative compartment in these baseline populations and a prospective series of polyp and control patients.

Patients and Methods

All patients were selected at colonoscopy. Polyp patients had one or more large-bowel adenomas more than 1 cm in diameter. Control patients were selected on the basis of a negative colonoscopy to the caecum, a normal double contrast barium enema and the absence of a family history of large-bowel neoplasia. To compare Brdu labelling throughout the large bowel, biopsies from ten adenoma patients and ten controls who were matched for sex and well matched for age were first obtained. Subsequently sigmoid biopsies were collected prospectively from a further 20 control and polyp patients, and the pattern of Brdu labelling was compared with those of the original populations to assess the sensitivity and specificity of the technique.

Biopsies obtained at colonoscopy were immediately established in organ culture [7]. Brdu was added to the culture medium at a final concentration of 100 μmol and labelling performed for 1 h prior to removal and fixation of the biopsies in Carnoy's fixative. Biopsies were processed to paraffin and 3-μm thick sections stained for incorporated Brdu using a standard avidin/biotin peroxidase technique. Forty axially sectioned hemi-crypts (crypt columns) were analysed per biopsy. For each crypt column the total number of cells and the number and position of Brdu-positive cells were directly keyed into a microcomputer for analysis. The LI (percentage of cells in S-phase) for each individual was determined from the percentage of Brdu-positive cells in each group of 40 crypt columns. All scoring was performed blind to the diagnosis of the patient.

To discriminate differences in the distribution of labelled cells within crypts, cumulative labelling distributions (CLDs) of Brdu-positive cells were generated. This method entails normalising each crypt column to a notional 100 cell positions, with cell position 0 at the crypt base and cell position 100 at the luminal surface. The distribution of positive cells is then expressed as a cumulative percentage for each crypt cell position centile. For example if a crypt column contains 20 cells and the 2nd, 4th, 6th and 10th cells from the bottom are labelled then these cells are assigned to the 10th, 20th, 30th, and 50th centiles of that crypt. The cumulative labelling corresponding to these centiles would then be 25%, 50%, 75% and 100% (Fig. 1). The results from all crypt columns in a sample are combined to generate a CLD. The CLD distributions of polyp and control patients were compared for each of the sites examined in the large bowel. Individual CLDs were subsequently generated for biopsies obtained prospectively and compared with the original sigmoid reference distributions to obtain a theoretical diagnosis for each patient examined.

Comparisons of LI were performed using Student's *t*-test. To test for significant differences between the CLDs of the reference populations a two-sample two-tailed Kolmogorov-Smirnov analysis was used. This non-parametric test defines a critical value "D" for any chosen probability at which the differences between cumulative distributions become significant. Differences between individual CLDs from the prospective series and the reference polyp and control distributions were tested by a one-sample Kolmogorov-Smirnov analysis, which defines a critical value D at which the null hypothesis that there is no difference between a test distribution and a theoretical one can be rejected.

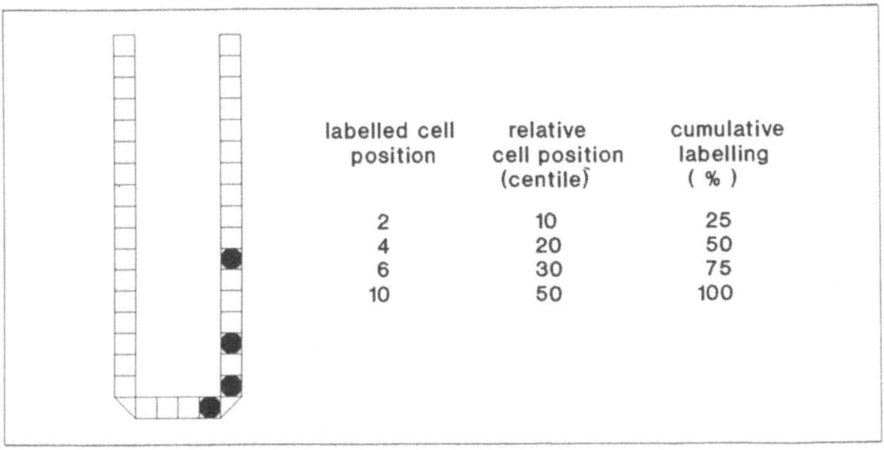

Fig. 1. Stylised crypt column demonstrating scoring of labelled cell positions and calculation of CLD in a crypt containing 20 cells

Table 1. Labelling index for individual regions within large intestine

Site	Polyp patients		Controls		*p*
	Mean	SEM	Mean	SEM	
Caecum	14.1	0.7	9.8	0.5	<0.001
Ascending	14.3	0.4	9.7	0.5	<0.001
Transverse	15.1	0.5	10.8	0.8	<0.001
Descending	15.6	0.8	11.3	0.5	<0.006
Sigmoid	14.9	0.8	10.3	0.5	<0.001
Rectum	14.2	0.6	11.8	0.6	<0.01

Results

Five male and five female subjects with a median age of 63 years (range 40–76) had adenomas present at colonoscopy. Controls were matched for sex and well matched for age (median 61 years, range 36–75). Overall percentage LI was higher in the large intestine of polyp patients than in the controls (mean 14.7 SEM 0.26 vs 10.64 SEM 0.25, $p < 0.001$). Mean LI for individual regions within the large intestine are summarised in Table 1. At each site examined the LI was significantly higher in the polyp patients. The CLDs obtained in the rectum are plotted in Fig. 2. In polyp patient mucosa it can be seen that the distribution is shifted towards the right of the X axis, i.e. there is a shift in the major zone of proliferation towards the luminal surface of the crypts. Thus in the rectum 100% labelling occurs by the 68th

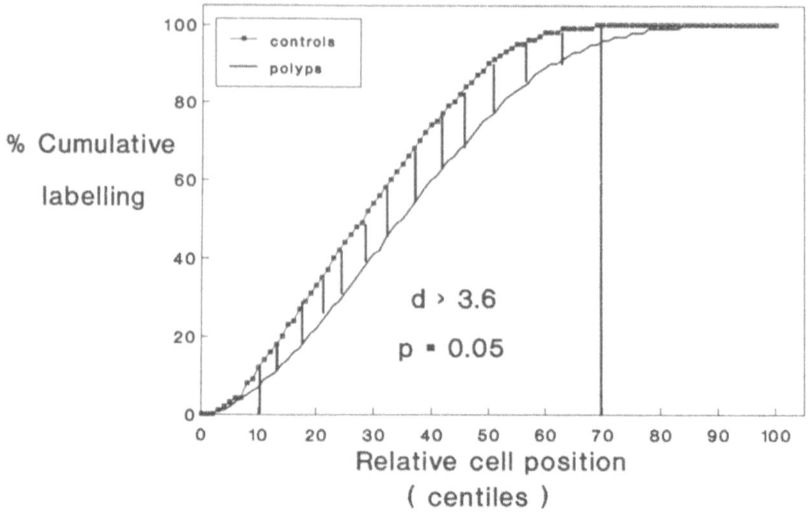

Fig. 2. CLDs in rectal mucosa of polyp and control patients. The curve is significantly shifted towards the right (i.e. the luminal surface of the crypts) in polyp-bearing mucosa. The *shaded area* represents the zone within the crypt where the upward shift in the proliferative compartment is significant ($p = 0.05$). d, critical D value

Table 2. Critical D values required in different regions of large intestine for an upward shift in polyp patients' CLDs to be significant and relative cell positions within crypts where shift is significant

Site	Critical D value[a]	Range where actual D > critical D value (centiles)
Caecum	3.6	13–62
Ascending	2.7	15–57
Transverse	3.5	19–55
Descending	3.4	20–56
Sigmoid	3.6	14–56
Rectum	3.6	9–70

[a] $p < 0.05$

centile in controls in contrast to the 84th centile in the polyp patients. The shaded area in the figure represents the zone within the crypt where this upward shift in the proliferative compartment is significant at a probability of 0.05. The critical D values at which an upward shift in the CLDs of the polyp patients becomes significant, and the relative cell positions within colonic crypts at which these D values are exceeded are listed in Table 2.

Prospective biopsies were obtained from a further eight male patients (median age 61 years, range 52–77) and 12 females (median age 63 years, range 30–85) who fulfilled the criteria of normal controls, and 12 male (median age 70 years, range 44–88) and eight females (median age 57 years, range 41–70) who had adenomas present at colonoscopy. Individual CLDs were tested for goodness of fit with each reference distribution, and the biopsy was then assigned as having a distribution of labelled cells compatible with and belonging to either the adenoma or control population. Analysis of the 20 biopsies from polyp patients correctly assigned 16 to the polyp group and three as controls; in one patient a diagnostic category could not be assigned due to the distribution being equally (and not significantly) different from both reference distributions. Similarily, of the 20 control patients, 17 were correctly assigned as controls and three as polyp patients, giving a sensitivity of 0.8, a specificity of 0.85 and a positive predictive value of 0.84.

Discussion

This is the first report of Brdu incorporation in biopsies taken throughout the large intestine and with this technique we have been able to confirm the findings of the only previous similar study performed with ^{3}H-T labelling and autoradiography [4]. These findings indicate the presence of abnormal proliferative activity throughout the large bowel of patients with adenomas which may be related to the recognised risk of metachronous and synchronous lesions in these patients.

It has been proposed that an early event in the development of colorectal tumours is the loss of ability of colonic epithelial cells to undergo terminal differentiation as they migrate up the crypt towards the luminal surface. This is reflected in a retained capacity to undergo DNA synthesis which leads to the presence of an expansion (stage 1) or a shift (stage 2) of the proliferative compartment towards the upper portions of the crypt [8]. Traditionally this shift in the distribution of the proliferative compartment has been analysed by dividing the crypts into several separate compartments with subsequent comparison of the LI between the different compartments [2–4, 8]. In this study an alternative method to describe the distribution of the proliferative compartment has been used, which allows the entire crypt to be analysed as a whole. When the distributions of the reference populations are compared there is a significant shift in the distribution of labelling in the polyp patients towards the luminal surface of the crypts which is significant throughout most of the major zone of proliferative activity i.e. the lower two thirds. This finding equates to the stage 1 and stage 2 proliferative defects described using traditional techniques. Furthermore the use of CLDs to analyse the proliferative compartment in individuals has been demonstrated to give an acceptable degree of sensitivity and specificity when tested in a prospective fashion, though it is likely that the power of the analysis could be further improved if the reference distributions were based on larger series of patients.

In conclusion we have found Brdu labelling in vitro, in conjunction with analyses of CLDs, to be a simple and rapid means of assessing proliferation in biopsies of large-bowel mucosa. This technique provides a sensitive "biomarker" of neoplasia in the assessment of high-risk populations and the effect of treatment strategies such as dietary intervention upon such populations.

References

1. Lipkin M (1988) Biomarkers of increased susceptibility to gastroin-testinal cancer: new application to studies of cancer prevention in human subjects. Cancer Res 48: 235–245
2. Lipkin M, Blattner WA, Gardner EJ, Burt RW, Lynch H, Deschner E, Winawer S, Fraumeni JF (1984) Classification and risk assessment of individuals with familial polyposis, Gardner's syndrome and familial non-polyposis colon cancer from [^{3}H] thymidine labeling patterns in colonic epithelial cells. Cancer Res 44: 4201–4207
3. Deschner EE, Lipkin M (1975) Proliferation patterns in colonic mucosa in familial polyposis. Cancer 35: 413–418
4. Terpstra OT, van Blankenstein M, Dees J, Eilers GA (1987) Abnormal pattern of cell proliferation in the entire colonic mucosa of patients with colon adenoma or cancer. Gastroenterology 92: 704–708
5. Lipkin M, Newmark H (1985) Effect of added dietary calcium on colonic epithelial-cell proliferation in subjects at high risk for familial colonic cancer. N Engl J Med 313: 1381–1384
6. Gratzner HG (1982) Monoclonal antibody to 5-Bromo and 5-Iododeoxyuridine: a new reagent for detection of DNA replication. Science 218: 474–475
7. Pritchett CJ, Senior PV, Sunter JP, Watson AJ, Appleton DR, Wilson RG (1982) Human colorectal tumours in short-term organ culture. Cell Tissue Kinet 15: 555–564
8. Deschner EE, Maskens AP (1982) Significance of the labeling index and labeling distribution as kinetic parameters in colorectal mucosa of cancer patients and DMH treated animals. Cancer 50: 1136–1141

Primary Malignant Lymphoma of the Rectum Associated with Chronic Ulcerative Colitis

A.L. Desai and P.G. Cassell

Introduction

Adenocarcinoma of the large bowel is well established as an important complication of chronic ulcerative colitis. The cumulative risk in patients with 25 years' history of extensive colitis is about 9% [1]. However, the relationship between long-standing ulcerative colitis and primary malignant lymphoma of the colon and rectum is not yet established because only a small number of cases have so far been reported. We report a case of Burkitt type high-grade non-Hodgkin's lymphoma in a patient with chronic ulcerative colitis.

Patient and Methods

A 53-year-old caucasian male patient was admitted to Wexham Park Hospital in September 1989 with 4 weeks' history of bloody diarrhoea, anaemia and weight loss. He was known to have ulcerative colitis of the whole colon and was first diagnosed in December 1984. Since then, he had been continuously on mesalazine, although he had required four short courses of oral steroids for acute exacerbations. Colonoscopy done in January 1988 had shown mild disease involving the entire length of the colon and multiple biopsies taken then had shown quiescent disease with mild mucosal dysplasia. At admission in September 1989, he had no superficial lymphadenopathy, abdominal examination was normal and rectal examination revealed a large tumour encircling the lower rectum with restricted mobility. The histological report on several biopsies from this lesion stated that there was infiltration of mucosa and submucosa by a monotonous population of pleomorphic lymphoid cells (lymphoblasts) with numerous scattered tingible body macrophages resulting in the so-called starry-sky appearance (Fig. 1). The cells showed intense positivity for leucocyte common antigen and light chain restriction with B-cell markers. The histological picture was thus of a high-grade non-Hodgkin's lymphoma with Burkitt type picture.

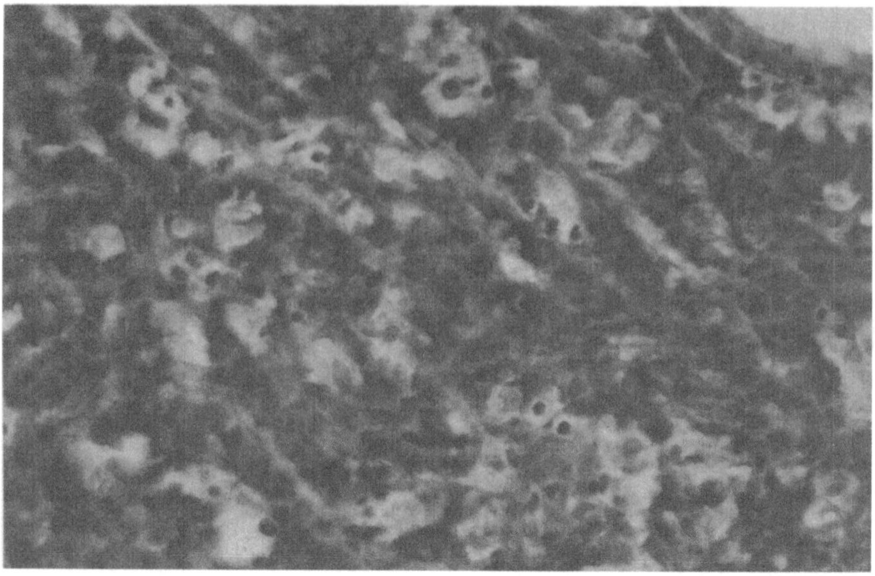

Fig. 1. Starry-sky, appearance of Burkitt type high-grade non-Hodgkin's lymphoma

The computed tomography (CT) scan showed a tumour extending from the rectosigmoid junction to anorectal region, but despite being extensive longitudinally, there was no infiltration into surrounding tissue planes (Fig. 2). The scan also demonstrated that the liver and the spleen were normal and that there was no lymphadenopathy in the abdomen or chest. His total and differential white cell count and bone marrow examination were normal.

In view of the aggressive histological picture and restricted mobility of the tumour, it was decided to refer the patient for chemotherapy in the first instance. He received vincristine, daunorubicin, asparaginase and prednisolone. In view of Burkitt type histology, 1 g cyclophosphamide was added to this regimen which lasted for 4 weeks. At week five, a further intensive chemotherapy including cytosine arabinoside and thioguanine was given. The cytopenia following both courses of chemotherapy was well tolerated. The patient's colitis had remained in complete remission during the period of chemotherapy presumably because of the steroids he was receiving as part of the chemotherapy. The oncologist's view at this stage was that the best chance of cure was to attempt high-dose chemotherapy and autologous bone marrow transplant and this was carried out in December 1989. He was also given a growth factor, growth colony-stimulating factor (G-CSF). Unfortunately, following this treatment he developed severe exacerbation of his ulcerative colitis. This was complicated by septicaemia, bone marrow suppression and also ventricular tachycardia due to cardio-

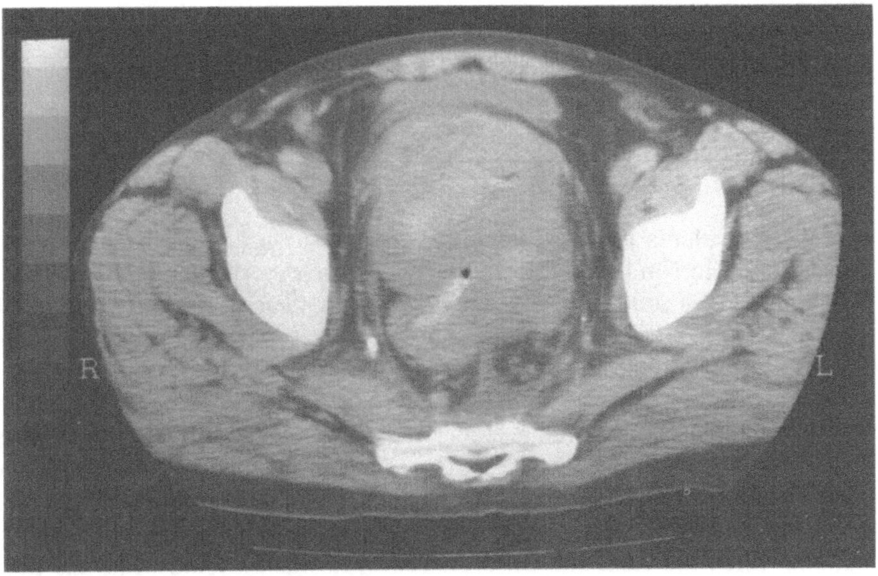

Fig. 2. CT Scan of pelvis showing a large rectal tumour

toxicity. Initially, because of bone marrow suppression, steroids were withheld but ultimately methyl prednisolone had to be given. Although this controlled his colitis, his bone marrow function never recovered and then he was found to have recurrent pelvic tumour. He died on 25th February, 1990.

Discussion

Primary malignant lymphoma of colon and rectum is extremely uncommon. In a large series of 4595 malignant tumours of colon reported from St. Mark's Hospital, London by Cornes et al. [2], only four cases of malignant lymphoma were found. Another series of 2510 malignant tumours of colon contained only 13 cases of malignant lymphoma [3]. Nugent et al. reported a series of 1313 resected specimens of large bowel with ulcerative colitis and found only five cases of malignant lymphoma [4], while a similar series of 352 resected specimens from St. Mark's Hospital showed only one case of malignant lymphoma (Table 1).

Malignant lymphoma is recognised as a complication of chronic inflammatory conditions of thyroid, lungs and salivary glands. Presumably, therefore, chronic inflammatory disease of the large intestine might be expected to give rise to malignant lymphoma. We found 29 cases of primary malignant lymphoma associated with ulcerative colitis reported in the literature. Out of

Table 1. Ulcerative colitis and malignant lymphoma

Resected specimens	Lymphoma	Percentage
1313	5	0.38
352	1	0.3

these, five patients also had adenocarcinoma of the large bowel. Dawson, Cornes and Morson [5] laid down five criteria to determine whether or not a lymphoma arose primarily within the bowel. In some of the cases previously reported, these criteria have not been strictly followed but this case satisfies these criteria completely.

Since Bargen [6] reported the first case in 1928, 28 further cases of primary malignant lymphoma associated with ulcerative colitis have been reported. However, the diagnosis of malignant lymphoma was made preoperatively in only two patients. We also established full histological diagnosis before the treatment was commenced. The average age of the patients when the tumour was first discovered was 47 years while the average duration of colitis was 11 years. All previously reported cases have been treated by radical surgery. In addition to surgery, four patients and adjuvant radiotherapy and chemotherapy while three patients had radiotherapy only. There were two perioperative deaths. Eight patients had recurrent disease within 12 months and two of these patients died within 12 months. Survival data are difficult to interpret, but it is clear that the three patients with long-reported disease-free survival received a combination of radical surgery, chemotherapy and radiotherapy.

A causal relationship between lymphoma and ulcerative colitis is still not proven. Cornes et al. suggested that repeated episodes of lymphoid hyperplasia associated with 25% of ulcerative colitis might lead to development of lymphoma [2]. Sataline suggested that the reticulo-endothelial system may play a significant role in pathogenesis of lymphoma [7]. Recently, seven previously reported cases have been immunohistologically studied [8] and this has shown that all these tumours had features of B-cell lymphoma, five out of seven tumours being high grade. All of them occurred at sites of involvement by colitis.

Conclusion

Evidence is emerging that links chronic ulcerative colitis to the development of primary malignant lymphoma. Preoperative diagnosis is important to lay out a management plan for these patients. The predominance of high-grade tumours suggests that the prognosis is poor and that carefully planned and radical treatment is needed to secure survivors. It appears that surgery together with radiotherapy and chemotherapy provides the best chance of a cure. On the basis of our experience and the literature review, we believe that surgery should precede adjuvant therapy. If, however, the tumour is fixed, then surgery should follow chemotherapy and/or radiotherapy.

References

1. Melville DM, Lennard-Jones JE, Morson BC, Ritchie JK, Williams CB (1988) Surveillance in extensive ulcerative colitis improves prognosis without always preventing cancer. Gut 29: A1494
2. Cornes JS, Smith JC, Southwood WF (1961) Lymphosarcoma in chronic ulcerative colitis with report of two cases. Br J Surg 49: 50–53
3. Warren S, Lulenski CR (1942) Primary solitary lymphoid tumors of gastro-intestinal tract. Ann Surg 115: 1–12
4. Nugent FW, Zuberi S, Bulan MB, Legg MA (1972) Colonic lymphoma in ulcerative colitis: report of four cases. Lahey Clin Found Bull 21: 104–111
5. Dawson IM, Cornes JS, Morson BC (1961) Primary malignant lymphoid tumours of the intestinal tract. Report of 37 cases with a study of factors influencing prognosis. Br J Surg 49: 80–89
6. Bargen JA (1928) Chronic ulcerative colitis complicated by malignant disease. Arch Surg 17: 561–576
7. Sataline LR, Mobley EM, Kirkham W (1963) Ulcerative colitis complicated by colonic lymphoma. Gastroenterology 44: 342–347
8. Shepherd NA, Hall PA, Williams GT, Codling BW, Jones EL, Levison DA, Morson BC (1989) Primary malignant lymphoma of the large intestine complicating chronic inflammatory bowel disease. Histopathology 15: 325–337

The Role of Colorectal Surgeons in the Treatment of Ovarian Carcinoma

N.A. Scott and P.F. Schofield

Introduction

Ovarian carcinoma will affect about 15 in every 1000 women in the United Kingdom in their lifetime [1]. Unfortunately the large majority of these patients (70%) will present with advanced disease – FIGO stages III and IV [2]. Cytoreductive surgery that results in a small tumour residuum, before initiating chemotherapy, is thought to improve chances of a patient with ovarian cancer obtaining a complete response [3].

Bilateral salpingo-oophorectomy, hysterectomy and omentectomy are accepted as being part of adequate cytoreductive surgery of ovarian cancer. However, intestinal resection and in particular colorectal resection may also be required to satisfactorily remove bulk pelvic disease [2, 3] We reviewed our experience of cytoreductive surgery in patients with ovarian cancer at the Christie Hospital. Our aim was to determine the importance of colorectal surgical skills to the optimal debulking of these tumours.

Methods and Patients

Patients with a diagnosis of ovarian carcinoma submitted to a laparotomy at the Christie Hospital between January 1987 and December 1989 were identified. The records of those patients undergoing primary cytoreductive surgery prior to chemotherapy were obtained. Patients with ovarian cancer undergoing surgery for complications of their disease (e.g. intestinal obstruction) or for a "second-look" procedure after chemotherapy were excluded.

Details recorded from the notes of the relevant patients included patient age, operability and the maximum transverse diameter (mm) of the largest residual disease after cytoreductive surgery. In particular the need for intestinal resection and intestinal stomas was noted. Postoperative morbidity and mortality within 30 days of surgery was also ascertained.

Results

Between January 1984 and December 1989 a total of 177 patients were referred to the Christie Hospital with a diagnosis of ovarian carcinoma (Fig. 1). Of these patients 58 (33%) had no bulk disease after previous surgery elsewhere; 66 (37%) had had an attempted debulking and 53 (30%) had only had their intra-abdominal disease biopsied. From January 1987 to December 1989, 28 of these patients, with evidence of residual bulk disease, were submitted to primary cytoreductive surgery prior to the initiation of chemotherapy.

Only four (14%) of the 28 patients were found to be inoperable. The remaining 24 (86%) patients were satisfactorily debulked. Six had no macroscopic residual disease at the end of this procedure and 18 were left with residual tumour nodules smaller than 5 mm in maximum transverse diameter after cytoreduction (Fig. 2).

All 24 debulked patients had bilateral salpingo-oophorectomy, hysterectomy and omentectomy. In addition 16 (67%) of these patients had an

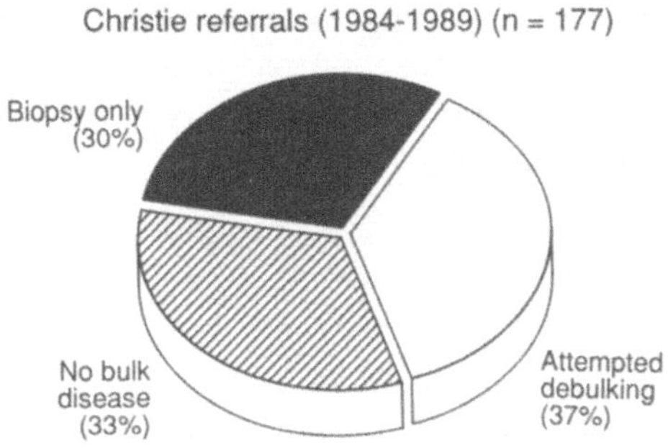

Fig. 1. Extent of ovarian cancer in patients referred to the Christie Hospital and Holt Radium Institute

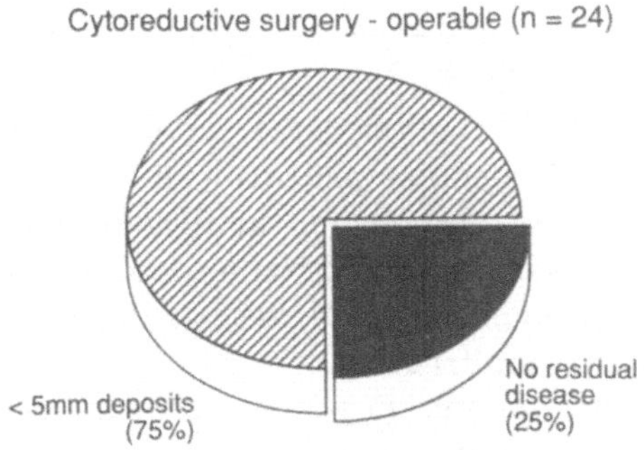

Fig. 2. Degree of cytoreduction achieved in the 24 operable patients

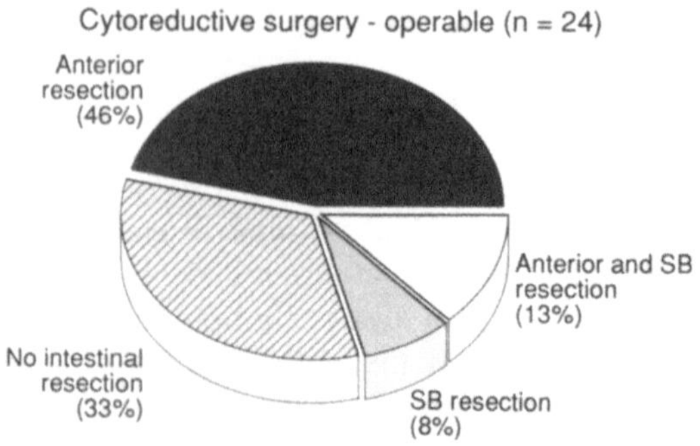

Fig. 3. Types of intestinal resection required to achieve optimal cytoreduction in the 24 operable patients. SB, small bowel.

intestinal resection. Small-bowel resection alone was performed in two (8%) patients, anterior resection alone in 11 (46%) patients and both anterior and small-bowel resection in three (13%) patients (Fig. 3). Thus a total of 14 (59%) patients required anterior resection of the rectum with primary reanastomosis to satisfactorily debulk their ovarian cancer. None of these patients required an intestinal stoma and none suffered a clinical anastomotic leak.

There were no deaths within 30 days of surgery. It is too early to present any details of long-term survival.

Discussion

The theoretical advantages of cytoreductive surgery in ovarian cancer include a reduction in the number of malignant cells by a factor of 1/1000 [4]. This reduces the chances of somatic mutations – that could result in drug resistance – occurring within the ovarian cancer cell population [4]. In addition the removal of large poorly vascularised tumour masses means that chemotherapy may be more effective against the smaller residual tumour nodules left after cytoreductive surgery [4].

Clinical studies have confirmed the survival advantages of debulking ovarian cancer and indicated that patients with residual tumour nodules less than 5 mm in transverse diameter do particularly well [5]. Cytoreductive surgery in this series was achieved down to residual tumour nodules of less than 5 mm transverse diameter in 24 patients or 86% of those undergoing laparotomy. This high incidence of optimal cytoreduction (86%) compares favourably with other reports, in which a similar degree of cytoreduction (i.e. <5 mm residual tumour nodules) was achieved in only 15% of patients operated on [5].

A particular difficulty encountered in achieving optimal cytoreduction of ovarian cancer is that of removing bulk pelvic disease that involves the rectum. In one series of 16 patients that could not be adequately debulked, nine (62%) had "large disease" in the pelvis; five of these nine patients had refused a colostomy preoperatively [5]. By contrast, we used anterior resection in 14 patients (59%) to remove bulk pelvic disease and so achieve an optimal level of cytoreduction.

Selecting and operating on patients with ovarian carcinoma to produce optimal cytoreduction involves a combination of clinical and surgical skills. In our experience a complete familiarity with anterior resection of the rectum was essential to successful cytoreduction without stomas and uncomplicated by anastomotic leaks. Ideally such skills would be available from a gynaecological oncologist [6, 7]. Until this ideal is readily available, a colorectal surgeon must be involved in the preoperative assessment and surgery of patients submitted to laparotomy for the cytoreduction of ovarian cancer.

References

1. Office of Population Censuses and Surveys (1981) Cancer statistics: incidence, survival and mortality in England and Wales. Stud Medical Popul Subj 43: 76–77
2. Piver MS (1987) Specialized surgery in ovarian cancer. Eur J Cancer Clin Oncol 23: 123–125
3. Wharton JT, Herson J (1981) Surgery for common epithelial tumors of the ovary. Cancer 48: 582–589
4. Richardson GS, Scully RE, Nikrui N, Nelson JH (1985) Common epithelial cancer of the ovary. N Engl J Med 312: 415–424
5. Hacker NF, Berek JS, Lagasse LD, Nieberg RK, Elashoff RM (1983) Primary cytoreductive surgery for epithelial ovarian cancer. Obstet Gynecol 61: 413–420
6. Lewis JL. The role of the gynecological oncologist. In Ballons S (ed) Gynecological oncology. Hall Medical, Boston, pp 6–7
7. Monaghan J (1987) Primary surgery discussion. In Sharp F, Soutter WP (eds) Ovarian cancer – the way ahead. Royal College of Obstetricians and Gynaecologists, pp 268–274

The Endoscopic Diagnosis of Anal Intra-Epithelial Neoplasia

J.H. Scholefield, C. Sonnex, I.C. Talbot, J.G. Palmer, A. Mindel and J.M. Northover

Introduction

The possible association between anal cancer and a sexually transmissible agent was first suggested from epidemiological data by Cooper in 1979 [1]. Other studies have supported this hypothesis; Austin [2] demonstrated an association between male homosexuality and anal cancer. Subsequently Daling [3] has demonstrated that receptive anal intercourse and genital warts are closely correlated with the subsequent development of anal cancer in males. Epidemiological studies of the aetiology of carcinoma of the uterine cervix have also suggested an association with a sexually transmissible agent. Common aetiological factors in tumours at these sites may reflect the common embryological origins of the anal and endocervical canals (both are derived from the cloacogenic membrane) [4]. Both the anal canal and the endocervical canal have squamous epithelium in their lower part and columnar epithelium above, with an area of transitional epithelium in between.

Recent molecular biological evidence has demonstrated an association between anal squamous cell carcinoma and human papillomavirus (HPV) type 16 [5]. This is the same virus, indeed the same HPV type, which has been associated with cervical cancer and with pre-malignant lesions of the cervix [6]. Extending this parallel, it might be expected that there may be clinically identifiable anal pre-malignant lesions similar to those identified on the cervix, and the identification of such lesions might lead to treatment to prevent the development of invasive cancer. This study addressed the first part of this hypothesis using an operating microscope to examine the microscopic anatomy of the anal canal. Histological examination and HPV typing (by DNA hybridisation) were performed on the biopsy specimens obtained during these examinations.

Methods

The boundaries of the anal canal and anal margin are poorly defined and vary from study to study. In the present study the boundaries of the anal canal have been defined as the area between the ano-rectal ring above and the junction with the perianal skin below; this latter being defined as the area which is visible on gentle retraction of the buttocks with the patient lying in the left lateral or lithotomy position.

A control group comprised 30 patients who had presented to a proctology out-patient department with anal fissure or fistula and who were examined under general anaesthesia prior to an elective operation for anal fistula or fissure. None of this group of patients had a previous history or clinical manifestations of anogenital HPV infection. All patients entered into this study were subjected to anal epithelial biopsy, histological examination and HPV DNA hybridisation.

The main study group comprised 85 patients who were attending a department of genitourinary medicine (71) with anal HPV infection or were referred to a proctology out-patient department with anal condylomata (14). None of these patients had been treated by application of podophyllin or similar mitogens in the previous 6 months. All patients entered into this study were subjected to biopsy of lesions, histological examination and HPV DNA hybridisations were performed on all biopsies.

Each patients was examined by naked eye and subsequently using an endoscope (the Zeiss OPM1 1FC colposcope) in conjunction with an oblique viewing proctoscope both before and after the application of a solution of 5% acetic acid to the epithelium in order to highlight HPV-infected and dysplastic areas of epithelium [7]. As on the cervix, 5% acetic acid causes a characteristic whitening of HPV-infected and dysplastic areas of epithelium. Acetic acid also highlights the appearance of the normal transitional zone. The criteria for the endoscopic diagnosis of intra-epithelial neoplasia of the cervix suggested by Reid et al. [7] were applied in the examination of the anal canal; they comprise a subjective assessment of the colour, vascular pattern, surface pattern and anatomical location of the lesion. These features give a guide to the likely histological diagnosis but histological examination remains the "gold standard" in the diagnosis of both anal intra-epithelial neoplasia (AIN) and cervical intra-epithelial neoplasia (CIN). Biopsies were taken from all abnormal areas seen endoscopically in the condyloma group and from the transition zone in the fistula and fissure group using a modified Ajax forceps under endoscopic control.

All anal biopsies were assessed histologically by one pathologist (ICT). The histological features of koilocytosis and parakeratosis were used to diagnose HPV infection in the biopsy specimens.

All the women in the main study group underwent cervical cytological assessment. Those women with abnormal cytology were referred for colposcopy and cervical biopsy.

DNA hybridisation studies were performed on 213 biopsy specimens from anal epithelium in all of the control group; for all dysplastic and all non-dysplastic anal lesions an alkaline hydrolysis method described by McIntyre and Stark [8] was used. This method has been adapted for use on formalin-fixed tissue by increasing the period of hydrolysis to 60 min in 0.4 *M* NaOH at 80°C [9]. HPV types 6, 11 and 16 DNA probes were used. These probes were radio labelled with [^{32}P] deoxycytidine triphosphate ([^{32}P] dCTP, 3000 Ci per mmol; Amersham, UK) by random priming [10] to a specific activity of 109 counts per cm^3. The HPV types 6b and 11 available for this study cross-hybridise even at high stringency; since infection with either type 6b or 11 cannot be distinguished, they are therefore referred to as 6/11. Southern blot analysis [11] was carried out where sufficient fresh tissue was available in order to validate the findings of the dot blot examinations (six of the dysplastic cases). All DNA hybridisations were performed on nylon membranes (Gene Screen Plus; New England Nuclear), at high stringency (0.5 *M* sodium phosphate at 72°C). Washing of membranes was carried out in 0.5x SSC, 0.1% sodium dodecyl sulphate (SDS) at 72°C. Autoradiography was performed on Kodak XAR 5 film between intensifying screens at −70°C for 24–72 h.

CIN is graded from I to III, according to the number of thirds of epithelial depth which appear dysplastic on histological section; thus in grade III the cells of the whole thickness of the epithelium appear dysplastic [12]. CIN III is equivalent to carcinoma in situ. A parallel grading of premalignant lesions in the anal canal, termed AIN, has been documented by Fenger [13] and has been used in the reporting of the anal lesions described here.

Human immunodeficiency virus (HIV) testing was performed using a competitive enzyme immuno assay (Wellcozyme); positive results were confirmed by antiglobulin enzyme-linked immunosorbent assay (ELISA, Abbott, UK) reverse antibody capture ELISA and gelatin particle agglutination assay.

Statistical evaluation of the results has been performed using a two-tailed Fisher exact test unless otherwise stated.

Results

In the control group of 30 patients in the haemorrhoid and anal fissure group (controls) 17 were men and 13 were women, (median age 38 years, range 16–60). These patients were examined whilst undergoing an anal operation for anal fistula or fissure; none had evidence of HPV infection or

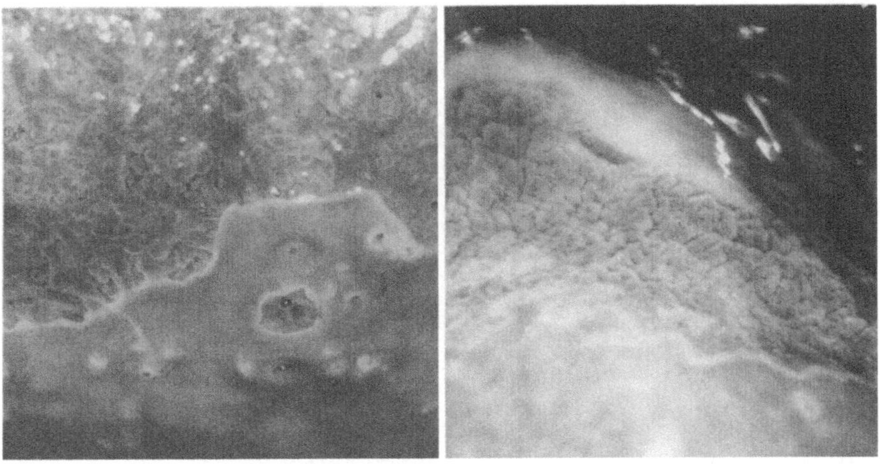

a b

Fig. 1a,b. The similarities of the cervical (**a**) and anal (**b**) transitional zones with columnar epithelium above and squamous epithelium below, with an area of transitional epithelium between

AIN either endoscopically or histologically. DNA hybridisation showed that none (0/30) of these patients had anal HPV infection.

The main study group comprised 85 patients; the median age was 30 years (range 17–58) and included 30 women and 55 men of whom 28 were homosexual. HIV antibody testing was performed on eight homosexual men after counselling. Six were found to be sero-positive and two were sero-negative. Twenty homosexual men declined testing.

There were strong similarities between the endoscopic appearances of the transitional zone in the anus and those described for the cervix (Fig. 1). Both lie between squamous and columnar epithelium and are of variable extent with an irregular proximal margin. Variation in the extent and morphology of the transitional zone has been demonstrated in resected anal canals both macroscopically and microscopically by Fenger [14].

AIN was diagnosed endoscopically in 21 of 85 patients with anal HPV infection. Eighteen of these were confirmed as dysplastic by histological examination. The remaining two showed evidence of koilocytosis without AIN. Five further cases of AIN which had been thought to be non-dysplastic condylomata endoscopically showed evidence of AIN on histological examination. In 18 of 23 dysplastic lesions the endoscopic and histological diagnoses were in agreement. The median age of the 23 patients with AIN was 27 years (range 19–58). These lesions are described in Tables 1–5.

Sixty-two patients with histologically confirmed anal HPV infection had no evidence of AIN histologically; there were 25 women, 11 homosexual men, and 26 heterosexual men. The median age of this group was 25 years

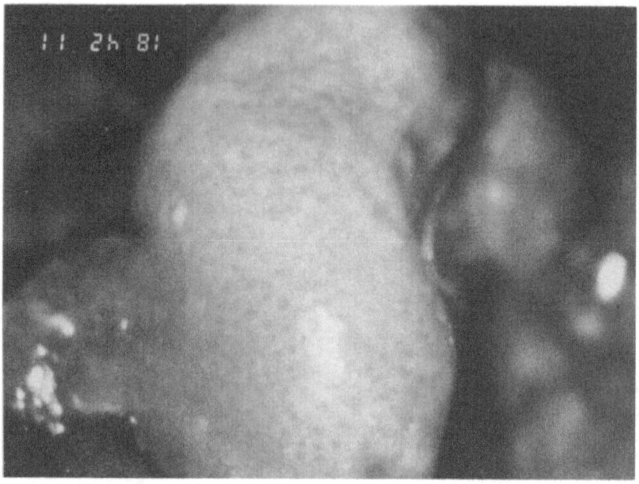

Fig. 2. An example of anal intra-epithelial neoplasia (AIN III) in the anal canal at the transitional zone; demonstrating the features of aceto-whitening, cobble-stoning and mosaicism

(range 18–52). These patients with non-dysplastic anal HPV infection are therefore well matched to the group with AIN.

Three out of four AIN III lesions were correctly diagnosed as dysplastic on endoscopy; but only six of ten AIN I lesions were diagnosed correctly on endoscopy. An example of AIN III is shown in Fig. 2; it demonstrates the features of irregular aceto-whitening, cobble-stoning and mosaicism and contains "corkscrew" vessels. In total there was histological evidence of AIN in 23 of 85 cases (27%) (Table 1). Of the 23 dysplastic lesions, 14 (68%) were located at the anal transition zone; (3/4AIN III, 6/9 AIN II, 5/10 AIN I lesions).

There was a statistically significant difference ($p = 0.01$) in the prevalence of AIN in the control group (0/20) compared to the prevalence of AIN in the wart virus-infected group (23/85).

In the main study group of 55 men, 1 of 27 (4%) heterosexual men with anal HPV infection had AIN, whereas 17 of 28 (61%) homosexual men with anal HPV infection had evidence of AIN ($p < 0.001$, Table 2). Six of the homosexual males in the study group were HIV antibody positive. All these patients had multiple condylomata. Three patients had focal AIN I and three more had AIN II (Table 3).

Of the 30 women in the study, ten had cytological evidence of CIN subsequently confirmed on biopsy. Five of ten (50%) of women in this group with evidence of CIA also had concurrent AIN (Table 1). There is a significant association between the observation of AIN in women with concurrent CIN ($p < 0.003$, Table 4).

Table 1. Details of patients with anal intra-epithelial neoplasia (AIN)

Age	Sex	Orientation	CIN	Endoscopy	Histology	HPV type
21	m	Heterosexual		Condyloma	AIN II	6
26	m	Homosexual		Dysplastic	AIN I	6
36	m	Homosexual		Condyloma	AIN I	6
26	m	Homosexual		Dysplastic	AIN I	6
25	m	Homosexual		Dysplastic	AIN I	6
40	m	Homosexual		Condyloma	AIN I	6
26	m	Homosexual		Dysplastic	AIN I	6
27	m	Homosexual		Condyloma	AIN I	6
24	m	Homosexual		Dysplastic	AIN I	6
28	m	Homosexual		Dysplastic	AIN II	6
33	m	Homosexual		Dysplastic	AIN II	6
27	m	Homosexual		Dysplastic	AIN II	6
28	m	Homosexual		Dysplastic	AIN II	16
26	m	Homosexual		Condyloma	AIN II	16
54	m	Homosexual		Dysplastic	AIN III	16
58	m	Homosexual		Dysplastic	AIN III	16
57	m	Homosexual		Dysplastic	AIN III	16
43	m	Homosexual		Dysplastic	AIN III	16
28	f		II	Dysplastic	AIN II	6 and 16
19	f		II	Dysplastic	AIN I	6
24	f		I	Dysplastic	AIN II	6
27	f		II	Dysplastic	AIN II	6
25	f		I	Dysplastic	AIN I	6

CIN, cervical intra-epithelial neoplasia; HPV, human papillomavirus; m, male; f, female

Table 2. The distribution of AIN in homosexual and heterosexual men[a]

	Homosexual	Heterosexual
AIN	17	1
No AIN (HPV infection)	11	26

[a] $p < 0.0001$ (Fisher exact test)

The distribution of HPV DNA types with respect to AIN is shown in Table 5. None of the AIN III lesions contained HPV 6/11, but all contained HPV type 16 DNA.

Discussion

The evidence of an aetiological role for HPV type 16 in the pathogenesis of cervical carcinoma is becoming more compelling. The association between anal squamous cell carcinoma and the same viral type is however less

Table 3. The distribution of AIN and HIV status in homosexual men[a]

	HIV + ve	HIV − ve/not tested
AIN	6	11
No AIN (HPV infection)	0	11

[a] $p = 0.055$ (Fisher exact test)

Table 4. The distribution of AIN and CIN in women[a]

	CIN	No CIN
AIN	5	0
No AIN (HPV infection)	5	20

[a] $p < 0.003$ (Fisher exact test)

Table 5. The distribution of HPV types and AIN lesions

	Controls Fissure/fistula ($n = 30$)	Main study group			
		HPV infection ($n = 62$)	AIN I ($n = 10$)	AIN II ($n = 9$)	AIN III ($n = 4$)
HPV 6/11 alone	0	51	10	6	0
HPV 16	0	8	0	2	4
HPV 6/11 and 16	0	3	0	1	0

well known. This series of cases of AIN is the first to be reported where endoscopic appearances, histology and DNA typing have been performed.

Apart from one study which reported two cases of "rectal dysplasia" [14], this study presents the first series of cases describing the endoscopic features of intra-epithelial neoplasia occurring in the anal canal.

Fenger [15] suggested a grading for AIN to parallel the grading of other genital pre-malignancies, and proposed that AIN may have a similar aetiology to other genital pre-malignancies. However his suggestion that endoscopic examination of the upper anal canal is not possible has been refuted by the present study. The whole length of the anal canal and the lower rectum can be adequately visualised using an operating microscope and biopsies of mucosa from these areas may be obtained under endoscopic guidance.

AIN arising in the anal canal has previously been thought to be a relatively uncommon lesion. Indeed, Fenger [15] described the incidence of (AIN) as an incidental histological finding in surgical specimens of anal epithelium as $0.2/10^5$ per year for the whole of Denmark. Only one of the 19 specimens in his series was found to be histologically condylomatous. The present study did not find histological evidence of AIN in any of the 20 patients with anal fissure or fistula, but there is a high prevalence of AIN in the patients with anal condylomata (28%).

This study has demonstrated a significantly higher prevalence of AIN in the homosexual men than in the heterosexual men studied ($p < 0.0001$). It has been suggested there may be subclinical immunosuppression in homosexual men [16], possibly due to the locally immunosuppressive effects of seminal plasma which are known to be rich in prostaglandins [17]. Such immunosuppression might make homosexual men more likely to develop AIN. Further studies are required to determine the significance of AIN and the risk of progression to invasive anal cancer. Since invasive anal cancer is much less common than invasive cervical cancer, one may postulate that the prevalence of AIN in the general population may be much lower than that found in this study of a highly selected population. An alternative explanation may be that the risk of progression from AIN to invasive cancer is lower for the anus than for the cervix. Reports from the United States suggest that there is an increasing incidence of anal cancer particularly in the anal canal [18] which may in part be attributable to the increasing prevalence of genital HPV infections.

The proportion of AIN which if left untreated would progress to invasive carcinoma and the time course over which such changes may occur are unknown. However, analogy with cervical pathology is probably relevant. In a prospective study of the progression of cervical lesions 85% of HPV 16 DNA positive women progressed from CIN I to CIN III in a 5-year period [19]. The evidence of progression from severe CIN to invasive cancer has been studied prospectively in only one series [20] in which 22% of those patients with persistent CIN III progressed to invasive cervical cancer within a follow-up period of 28 years.

In the present study the AIN I and AIN II lesions occurred in the younger end of the age range of the main study group (median 26 years; range 19–43). All the AIN III lesions occurred in patients who were over the age of 40 years (median 55.5 years; range 43–58). All four of the AIN III lesions contained HPV type 16 DNA. An interesting analogy with cervical dysplasia is the suggestion that there may be an association between the more severe grades of CIN, HPV type 16 infection and increasing age [21].

The prevalence of anal dysplastic lesions in HIV positive homosexuals was greater than in the group of homosexual males who were HIV negative or "not known" to be HIV positive. However, the data do not achieve statistical significance ($p = 0.055$). This comparison is likely to be of limited value as some of those individuals of unknown HIV antibody status are likely to be HIV antibody positive.

It is interesting that all the AIN III lesions contained HPV type 16 DNA whereas all of the AIN I lesions contained HPV type 6/11 DNA only. HPV type 16 DNA was identified in 7 of 23 (30%) of the dysplastic lesions. Though this is a small series these findings suggest that the distribution of HPV types in anal pre-malignancies are similar to those seen in the cervical pre-malignancies. The HPV types in the non-dysplastic condylomatous lesions were predominantly 6/11 (87%); HPV type 16 DNA was found in 11 of 62 (18%) of this group of patients. There is no significant difference in the prevalence of HPV type 16 infection in the dysplastic group compared with the non-dysplastic condylomata ($p > 0.3$). Not all patients with HPV type 16 infection have AIN. Further prospective studies are being undertaken to determine the prevalence of anal HPV infections and the natural history of these infections.

Several studies have estimated the prevalence of HPV type 16 infection of the cervix; their results range from 5% to 80% in normal cervices. The large variation in these estimates is in part explained by the advent of the polymerase chain reaction [22]. This confusing picture has recently been compounded by the finding that there may be subtypes of HPV type 16 which may have differing oncogenic potential [23]. Further studies are awaited with interest.

The prevalence of AIN in condylomatous lesions reported in the present study is 27%. This may be partly explained by the number of homosexual males seen (28), 17 of 28 (61%) of whom had evidence of AIN. The high incidence of AIN in homosexuals (both HIV antibody positive and negative) has previously been reported as an observation on cytological and histological specimens but not diagnosed endoscopically [24, 25]. These results are similar to the prevalence of AIN reported in a series of predominantly homosexual patients with anal condylomata in which the proportion with dysplasia was 30% [26].

The observation that 68% of the AIN lesions were in the anal transitional zone may suggest that HPV infections in this area are more susceptible to dysplastic change than infections at the anal margin. Follow-up of these lesions is being undertaken in order to determine their natural history.

Multifocal female genital tract intra-epithelial neoplasia is more frequently recognised as increasing evidence to suggest that the anal, vulval and vaginal epithelium may be susceptible to the development of HPV-related AIN in much the same manner as the cervix [14]. A previous report of multifocal genital intra-epithelial neoplasia described two cases of "rectal intra-epithelial neoplasia" in a woman with co-existent CIN [14]. In the present study it has been noted that the transitional zone is variable in extent from patient to patient, confirming the observations of Fenger [15]. This is important as a wide transformation zone could lead to the mistaken diagnosis of squamous metaplasia of the rectal epithelium in some instances. Squamous metaplasia in the rectum is a very rare condition [27]. Perhaps, in retrospect those lesions previously called "rectal" dysplasia were situated in the anal transitional zone rather than in the rectum.

In conclusion, the anal canal can be examined using an operating microscope and dysplastic lesions identified. Further detailed prospective studies on the natural history of AIN are required. Furthermore, this study has demonstrated that there is an association between concurrent CIN and AIN. This supports the hypothesis that the anal and cervical epithelium are susceptible to similar carcinogens.

References

1. Cooper HS, Patchefsky AS, Marks G (1979) Cloacogenic carcinoma of the anorectum in homosexual men: an observation of four cases. Dis Colon Rectum 22: 557–558
2. Austin DF (1982) Etiological clues from descriptive epidemiology: squamous carcinoma of the rectum or anus. NCI Monogr 62: 89–90
3. Daling JR, Weiss NS, Hislop TG, Maden C, Coates RJ, Sherman KJ, Ashley RL, Beagrie M, Ryan JA, Corey L (1987) Sexual practices, sexually transmitted diseases and the incidence of anal cancer. N Engl J Med 317: 973–977
4. Cabrera A, Tsukada Y, Pickren JW, Moore R, Bross ID (1966) Development of lower genital carcinomas in patients with anal carcinoma. A more than casual relationship. Cancer 19: 470–480
5. Palmer JG, Shepherd NA, Jass JR, Crawford LV, Northover JM (1987) Human papillomavirus type 16 DNA in anal squamous cell carcinoma. Lancet ii: 42
6. Reid R, Stanhope CR, Herschman BR, Booth E, Phibbs GS, Smith JP (1982) Genital warts and cervical cancer. I. Evidence of an association between subclinical papillomavirus infection and cervical malignancy. Cancer 50: 377–387
7. Reid R, Stanhope CR, Herschman BR, Crum CP, Agronow SJ (1984) Genital warts and cervical cancer. IV. A colposcopic index for differentiating subclinical papillomaviral infection from cervical intraepithelial neoplasia. Am J Obstet Gynecol 149: 815–823
8. McIntyre P, Stark GR (1988) A quantitative method for analyzing specific DNA sequences directly from whole cells. Anal Biochem 174: 209–214
9. Scholefield JH, McIntyre P, Palmer JG, Coates PJ, Shepherd NA, Northover JM (1990) DNA hybridisation of routinely processed tissue for detecting HPV DNA in anal squamous cell carcinomas over 40 years. J Clin Pathol 43: 133–136
10. Feinberg AP, Vogelstein B (1983) A technique for radiolabeling DNA restriction endonuclease fragments to high specific activity. Anal Biochem 132: 6–13
11. Reed KC, Mann DA (1985) Rapid transfer of DNA from agarose gels to nylon membranes. Nucleic Acids Res 13: 7207–7221
12. Richart RM (1973) Cervical intraepithelial neoplasia. Pathol Annu 8: 301–328
13. Fenger C (1978) The anal transitional zone. Acta Pathol Microbiol Scand [A] 86: 225–230
14. McCance DJ, Clarkson PK, Dyson JL, Walker PG, Singer A (1985) Human papillomavirus types 6 and 16 in multifocal intraepithelial neoplasias of the female lower genital tract. Br J Obstet Gynecol 92: 1093–1100
15. Fenger C, Thue Nielsen V (1986) Intraepithelial neoplasia in the anal canal. The appearance and relation to genital neoplasia. Acta Pathol Microbiol Immunol Scand [A] 94: 343–349
16. Frazer IH, MacKay IR, Crapper RM, Jones B, Gust ID, Sarngadharan MG, Campbell DC, Ungar B (1986) Immunological abnormalities in asymptomatic homosexual men: correlation with antibody to HTLV-III and sequential changes over two years. Q J Med 61: 921–933

17. Saxena S, Jha P, Farooq A (1985) Immunosuppression by human seminal plasma. Immunol Invest 14: 255–269
18. Wexner SD, Milsom JW, Dailey TH (1987) The demographics of anal cancers are changing. Identification of a high-risk population. Dis Colon Rectum 30: 942–946
19. Campion MJ, McCance DJ, Cuzick J, Singer A (1986) Progressive potential of mild cervical atypia: prospective cytological, colposcopic, and virological study. Lancet ii: 237–240
20. McIndoe WA, McLean MR, Jones RW, Mullins PR (1984) The invasive potential of carcinoma in situ of the cervix. Obstet Gynecol 64: 451–458
21. Meanwell CA, Cox MF, Blackledge G, Maitland NJ (1987) HPV 16 DNA in normal and malignant cervical epithelium: implications for the aetiology and behaviour of cervical neoplasia. Lancet i: 703–707
22. Young LS, Bevan IS, Johnson MA, Blomfield PI, Bromidge T, Maitland NJ, Woodman CB (1989) The polymerase chain reaction: a new epidemiological tool for investigating cervical human papillomavirus infection. Br Med J 298: 14–18
23. Tidy JA, Vousden KH, Farrell PJ (1989) Relation between infection with a subtype of HPV 16 and cervical neoplasia. Lancet i: 1225–1227
24. Croxson T, Chabon AB, Rorat E, Barash IM (1984) Intraepithelial carcinoma of the anus in homosexual men. Dis Colon Rectum 27: 325–330
25. Frazer IH, Medley G, Crapper RM, Brown TC, MacKay IR (1986) Association between anorectal dysplasia, human papillomavirus, and human immunodeficiency virus infection in homosexual men. Lancet ii: 657–660
26. Syrjänen SM, von Krogh G, Syrjänen KJ (1989) Anal condylomas in men. 1. Histopathological and virological assessment. Genitourin Med 65: 216–224
27. Morson BC, Dawson IM (1979) Gastrointestinal Pathology. Blackwell, London

Tracking the Familial Adenomatous Polyposis Gene Carriers by Indirect Ophthalmoscopy

F. Munier, J.-C. Givel, L. Zografos and P.-A. Grounauer

Introduction

Familial adenomatous polyposis (FAP) is an autosomal-dominant disease with delayed expression, in which multiple polyps develop throughout the colon with a malignant potential of 100%. Genetic counselling and follow-up of patients at risk is essential for presymptomatic diagnosis. Prophylaxis of cancer arising from this condition would greatly improve if a genetic or a congenital phenotypic marker of gene carriers were available.

In 1935, Cabot and associates first described "several punctate pigmented areas in fundi" in a patient with Gardner's syndrome [4]. These pigmented spots were later histologically documented as congenital hypertrophy of the retinal pigment epithelium (Chrpe) [3]. Ophthalmoscopically Chrpe is characterized by isolated round or ovoid hyperpigmented lesions. The clinical significance of bilateral and multiple foci of Chrpe in connection with Gardner's syndrome was recognized by Blair and Trempe in 1980 [2].

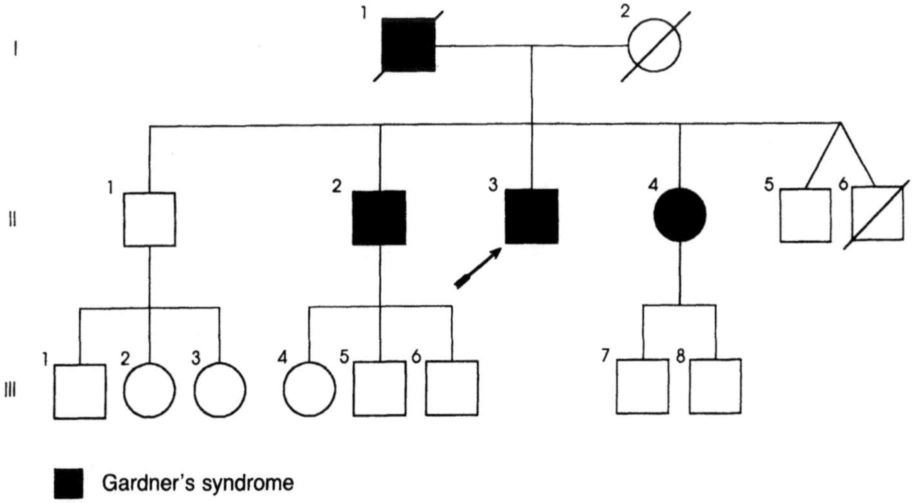

Fig. 1. Pedigree of the family with Gardner's syndrome

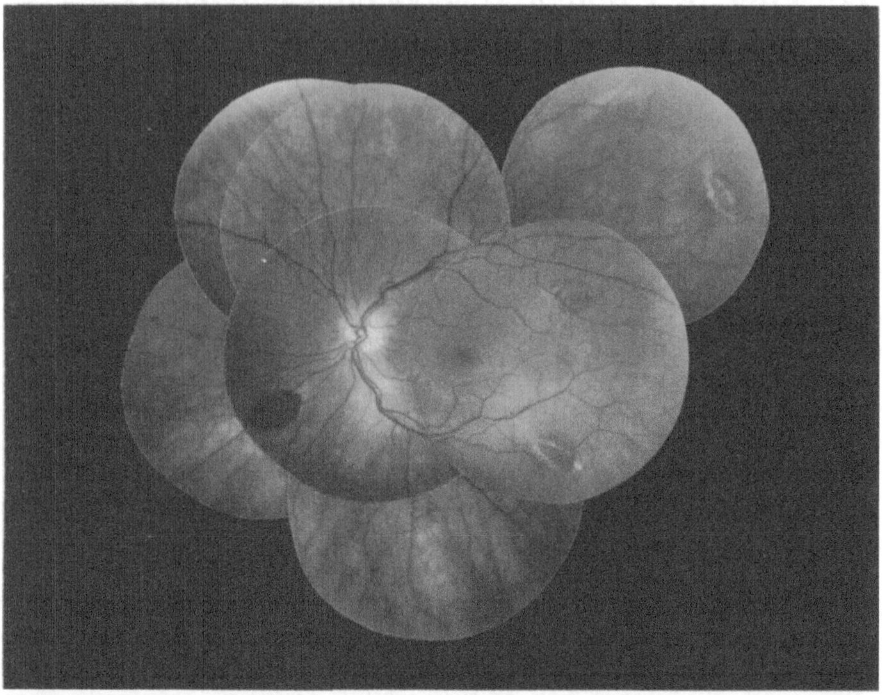

a

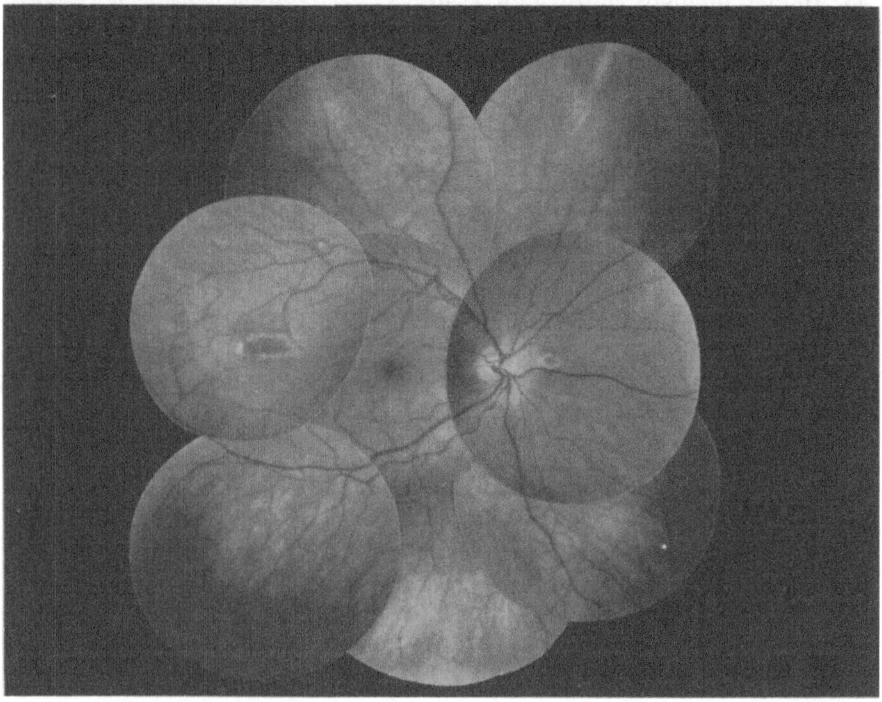

b

Fig. 2a–d. Proband's fundi. **a,b** Photographs of posterior pole and midperiphery of the retina, and **c,d** drawings of both posterior and peripheral lesions

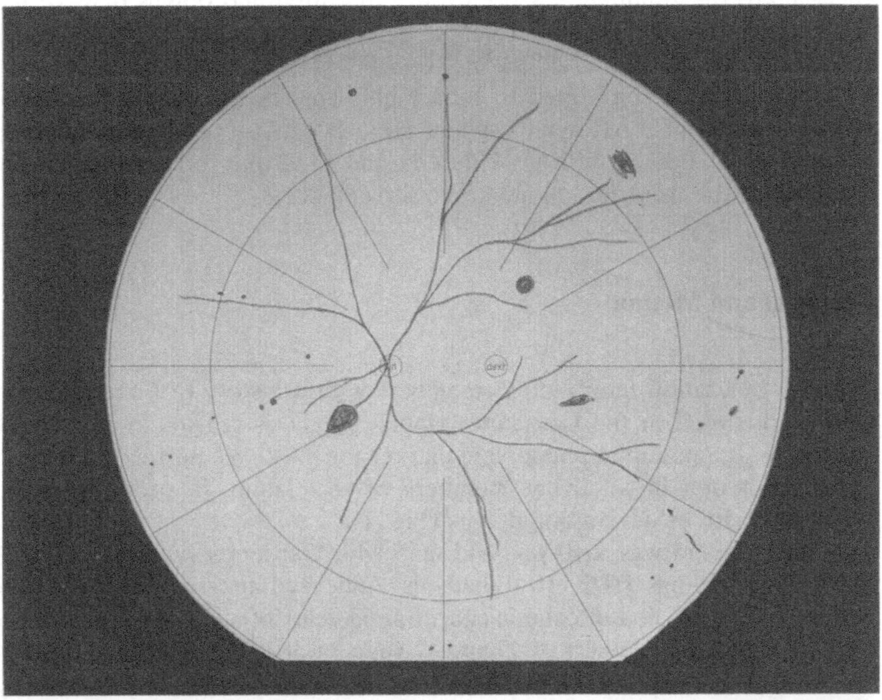

c

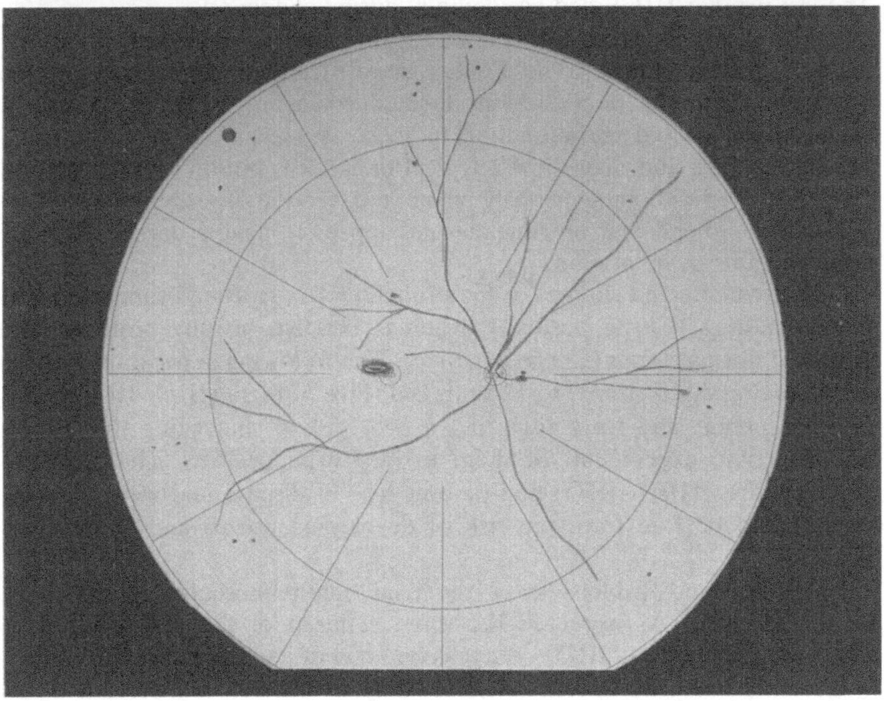

d

Since then, the simultaneous occurrence of Chrpe and polyps of FAP was ascertained through ophthalmoscopic screening of affected pedigrees [1, 5–11].

Chrpe is now considered to be a highly specific (95.2%) and sensitive (78%) marker of FAP gene carriers [10]. It can be used to predict the occurrence of polyps in FAP kindreds and thus may provide supportive evidence of the need for colonoscopic surveillance.

Material and Method

A three-generation family of 16 members with a history of Gardner's syndrome, recorded in the Lausanne familial polyposis registry, was assessed for Chrpe as a potential phenotypic marker for FAP. We performed indirect ophthalmoscopy in all living members of this family in order to detect patients at risk of developing polyps (Fig. 1).

The proband was a 40-year-old man with Gardner's syndrome (Fig. 1, II/3). Two siblings (II/2, II/4) had also inherited the disease from their father (I/1), who died of colonic cancer at 63 years of age. The proband had two other healthy brothers of 45 and 42 years of age (II/1, II/5), who had no extracolic manifestation of Gardner's syndrome and negative colonoscopy. The last brother (II/6) died accidentally during childhood.

Figure 2a,b show the pathognomonic picture of the proband's fundi with multiple foci of Chrpe. The lesions are distributed throughout all four quadrants, with the larger lesions located posteriorly (Fig. 2a,b) and the smaller ones located peripherally (Fig. 2c,d). Posterior lesions are ovoid to oblong in shape and they show a typical radial distribution around the optic disk; they are nonhomogeneously pigmented. On the other hand, peripheral lesions are either linear or punctate and appear to have a darker and more homogeneous pigmentation.

The two affected siblings of the proband (II/2, II/4) had similar bilateral ocular findings (Chrpe positive), whereas the two healthy brothers (II/1, II/5) had normal fundi (Chrpe negative). The following generation involved eight children aged from 7 to 17 years old. Five of them (III/4–III/8) had an affected parent and were thus had a 50% risk of inheriting the disease. So one could expect half of them to be Chrpe positive. The remaining three children (III/1–III/3) had parents free of disease and were therefore expected to be free from the risk of developing polyps and to be Chrpe negative.

Figure 3 and Table 1 show the final ophthalmoscopic results of the whole pedigree. As expected the three children of the first kindred are Chrpe negative (III/1–III/3), whereas one boy of each of the other kindreds was found to be Chrpe positive (III/5, III/8), and therefore a presumed gene carrier of Gardner's syndrome.

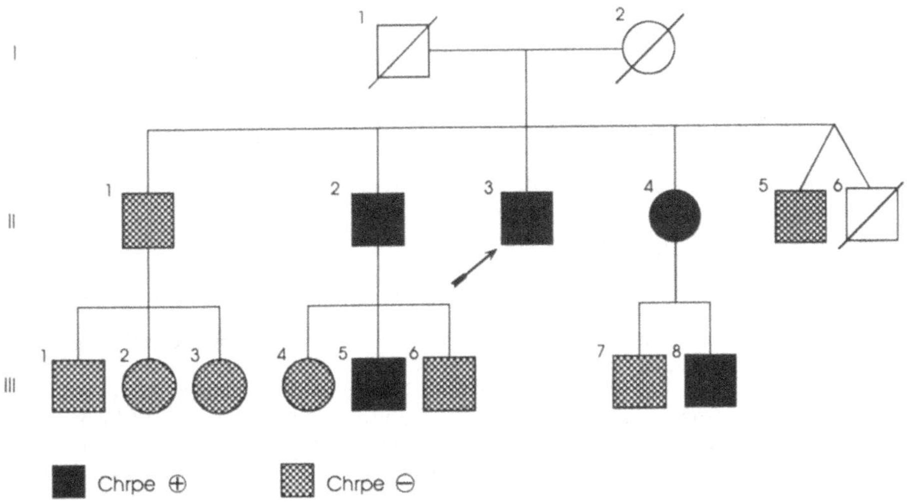

Fig. 3. Final ophthalmoscopic results in the family with Gardner's syndrome

Table 1. Total number of fundus lesions in family with Gardner's syndrome

Family member	Total number of fundus lesions
II/2	11
II/3	47
II/4	33
III/5	9
III/8	12

Discussion and Conclusion

We have recommended that colonoscopy should be performed regularly in the two Chrpe-positive children, but this has not been done up to now. On the other hand, it seems reasonable to perform colonoscopy less frequently in Chrpe-negative patients. We know from the literature that Chrpe is present in two thirds of FAP families and is pathognomonic of the disease whether multifocal (⩾4 spots) or bilateral [8].

The search for Chrpe is an inexpensive and non-invasive procedure which is very specific although less sensitive. Furthermore Chrpe is thought to be of congenital origin. In our opinion, indirect ophthalmoscopy should form part of the initial investigation in FAP patients and should also be extended to first-degree relatives of patients who are Chrpe positive.

References

1. Berk T, Cohen Z, McLeod RS, Parker JA (1988) Congenital hypertrophy of the retinal pigment epithelium as a marker for familial adenomatous polyposis. Dis Colon Rectum 31: 253–257
2. Blair NP, Trempe CL (1980) Hypertrophy of the retinal pigment epithelium associated with Gardner's syndrome. Am J Ophthalmol 90: 661–667
3. Buettner H (1975) Congenital hypertrophy of the retinal pigment epithelium. Am J Ophthalmol 79: 177–189
4. Cabot RC (1935) Case records of the Massachusetts General Hospital: case 21061. N Engl J Med 212: 263–267
5. Diaz-Llopis M, Menezo JL (1988) Congenital hypertrophy of the retinal pigment epithelium in familial adenomatous polyposis. Arch Ophthalmol 106: 412–413
6. Lewis RA, Crowder WE, Eierman LA, Nussbaum RL, Ferrell RE (1984) The Gardner syndrome. Significance of ocular features. Ophthalmology 91: 916–925
7. Lyons LA, Lewis RA, Strong LC, Zuckerbrod S, Ferrell RE (1988) A genetic study of Gardner syndrome and congenital hypertrophy of the retinal pigment epithelium. Am J Hum Genet 42: 290–296
8. Romania A, Zakov ZN, McGannon E, Schroeder T, Heyden F, Jagelman DG (1989) Congenital hypertrophy of the retinal pigment epithelium in familial adenomatous polyposis. Ophthalmology 96: 879–884
9. Stein EA, Brady KD (1988) Ophthalmologic and electro-oculographic findings in Gardner's syndrome. Am J Ophthalmol 106: 326–331
10. Traboulsi EI, Krush AJ, Gardner EJ, Booker SV, Offerhaus GJ, Yeardley JH, Hamilton SR, Luk GO, Giardiello FM, Welsh SB, Hughes JP, Maumenee IH (1987) Prevalence and importance of pigmented ocular fundus lesions in Gardner's syndrome. N Engl J Med 316: 661–667
11. Traboulsi EI, Maumenee IH, Krush AJ, Giardiello FM, Levin LS, Hamilton SR (1988) Pigmented ocular fundus lesions in the inherited gastrointestinal polyposis syndromes and in hereditary nonpolyposis colorectal cancer. Ophthalmology 95: 964–969

Part III: Inflammatory Bowel Diseases

The Role of Intestinal Microbes in Ulcerative Colitis: Studies on the Rectal Mucosa-Associated Microflora

M.G. Hartley, M.J. Hudson, M.J. Hill, A.E. Gent, R.H. Grace, M.D. Hellier and E.T. Swarbrick

Introduction

There is broad agreement that microbes play an important role in the aetiology and pathogenesis of ulcerative colitis (UC), probably via an abnormal local immune response to one or several microbial antigens or metabolites; this is clearly in addition to their role in local tissue invasion and microabscess formation. However, numerous investigations have failed to identify either an aetiological agent or a consistent alteration in the composition or balance of the complex faecal microflora.

During the past 3 years we have re-examined the role of intestinal microbes in UC in two separate but linked studies. Firstly, we sought enteric pathogens in the faeces of 95 patients at initial diagnosis and after treatment for newly diagnosed UC. Secondly, we characterised the microflora intimately associated with the intestinal mucosa; since the lesions of UC are confined to the colorectal mucosa, we argued that a study of pathogenic or protective effects of the mucosa-associated flora (MAF) would be of greater relevance due to its unique anatomical position in contrast to investigation of faecal or luminal microflora.

Results

Despite using sensitive techniques for the recovery of the "new" enteric pathogens (*Campylobacter*, *Yersinia*, etc.) bacterial pathogens were not found in our survey of 95 patients with UC, although a single patient had a cryptosporidial infestation. Interestingly, the faeces of six patients contained a cytotoxin, the identity of which is the subject of further investigation.

We have isolated and characterised the MAF of rectal biopsy tissue samples taken from the following patient groups:

1. Thirty patients with active UC but without previous history, studied at presentation and after 3 and 12 weeks treatment
2. Twenty patients with UC in relapse, studied at presentation and after 3 and 12 weeks of treatment
3. Sixty-six patients with UC in remission
4. Nine patients from the quiescent UC group (3.), studied during a subsequent relapse of their disease
5. Fifteen patients without inflammatory bowel disease, included as a control group

The MAF was estimated and characterised using quantitative microbiological techniques suitable for the recovery of the fastidious anaerobic bacteria found in the colon. Bacterial counts were expressed as $\log_{10}$ bacteria/g tissue and compared by appropriate parametric and non-parametric statistical methods. An index of clinical severity was compiled for each patient at each visit. Samples of serum taken at each visit were stored for later analyses. Representative bacterial isolates from each sample were also stored frozen for subsequent studies.

The MAF was simpler than the faecal flora from which it is largely derived. The predominant flora was obligately anaerobic and comprised bacteroides, bifidobacteria and gram-positive cocci. The most common facultatives were enterococci; indeed, only 39% of our patients with active, untreated new disease had detectable numbers of *Escherichia coli* in the rectal MAF.

There was considerable inter-patient variability in total and differential counts; this is similar to the variation seen in the faecal microflora. The total counts ranged from less than 3.0/g to 8.29/g. Statistical comparisons of counts and carriage rates showed active UC was associated with significant reductions in counts of total flora, anaerobes including bifidobacteria, eubacteria, clostridia and facultatives including lactobacilli and enterobacteria. The carriage rates of enterobacteria, clostridia and bifidobacteria were also markedly reduced in active disease; for bifidobacteria, this trend was reversed during treatment.

Previous studies by other workers on isolates from faecal flora have incriminated *E. coli* as playing a possible role in the pathogenesis of UC, either by alterations in counts or pathogenic properties, as detected by such markers as haemolysin production and adhesion to cell lines. In addition to the low counts of *E. coli* in the MAF, our UC patient isolates were neither significantly more adhesive to cell lines nor more hydrophobic than those from control patients. We are currently studying this observation in more detail.

In order to minimise the statistical difficulties due to inter-patient variability, the data from individual patients was re-analysed for microbiological changes in the MAF with respect to their clinical response. We found consistent alterations were confined to both the absolute and proportional counts of the strictly anaerobic gram-positive cocci (AnGPC). This has not been reported previously in microbiological studies of UC and dictates the direction of our future studies. The AnGPC are a poorly defined group of bacteria, comprising at least six genera. The AnGPC include some species which are extremely oxygen sensitive and possess the ability to break down biopolymers such as mucins and complex carbohydrates; others are well-documented pathogens of man, particularly in mixed sepsis. We will study our isolates for such metabolic activities and examine the nature of the immune response mounted against them, using our stored serum samples.

Epidemiology and Clinical Course of Patients with Crohn's Disease at a Central Surgical University Clinic in Switzerland (1973–1985)

H. STRIFFELER, W. SCHWEIZER and M. GILG

Introduction

Forty-five years after the first description of Crohn's disease the interval from first symptoms to diagnosis is still approximately 3 years and in spite of better knowledge and better diagnostic facilities the aetiology and prognosis in the individual case is still unpredictable. Because of the considerable effort required [1–4], epidemiological studies are few, although they may help to increase our understanding of the disease. We therefore carried out a retrospective survey of our patients with respect to epidemiology, aetiology, the clinical course of the disease and the patient's employment status.

Patients and Methods

We analysed retrospectively 108 patients with Crohn's disease admitted to the Department of Visceral and Transplantation Surgery of the Central University Hospital, Inselspital Bern, during the period from January 1973 to December 1985. The mean time of observation following appearance of the first symptoms was 13 years (range 1–39 years). All interviews and the review of medical histories were conducted by one examiner using a standardized questionnaire. Patients with typical clinical features of Crohn's disease but an unclear histological finding were excluded from the study. Many patients were referred from other departments of our hospital or from other hospitals to our clinic because of complications of Crohn's disease and represent therefore a selected group of surgical Crohn's disease patients within a Central University Hospital. On the basis of other epidemiological studies and the referral pattern in Switzerland we may assume that our patients represent about one-third of the Crohn's disease patients in an area of about one million inhabitants [1–5].

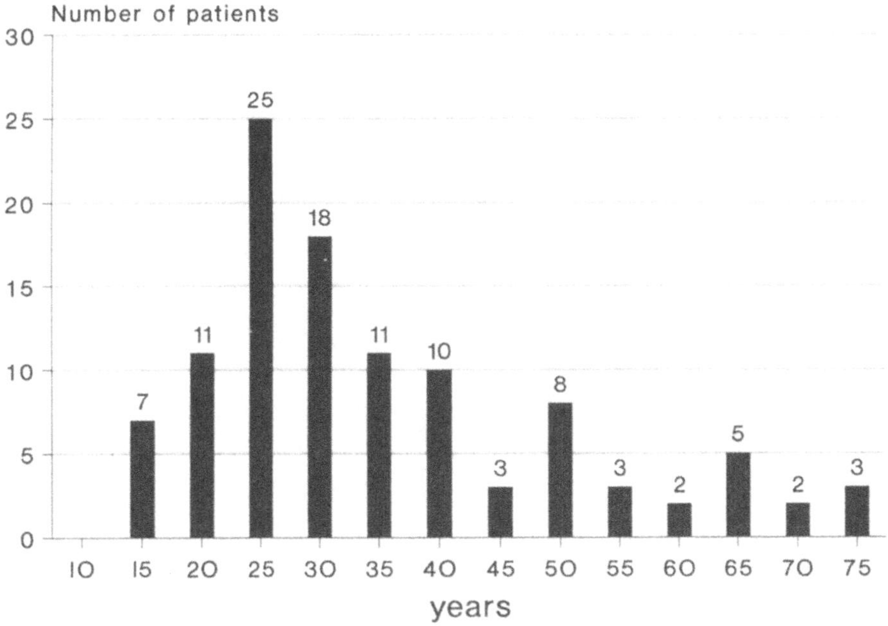

Fig. 1. Age at onset of first symptoms of Crohn's disease

Results

We evaluated 108 patients (57% male, 43% female) with a mean age at appearance of the first symptoms before diagnosis of 32 years (range 10–73 years). Eight per cent of our patients had one first-degree relative also suffering from Crohn's disease. The highest incidence of onset of Crohn's disease was found at between 20 and 25 years of age, with 23% of all patients falling in this group. A second peak around 60 years of age was not seen. The duration of the symptoms before diagnosis varied from 0 to 25 years with a mean of 3.2 years. Fifty-seven per cent of our patients developed the disease before their 30th year, and 17% before their 20th year. After the age of 50 only 14% of the patients developed Crohn's disease (Fig. 1).

Of the 46 female patients, 28 had had at least one pregnancy. In only two patients were repeated attempts to become pregnant not followed by pregnancy. One of the women had suffered from Crohn's disease for 16 years, the other for 4 years. All the men with Crohn's disease who wished to have children were able to do so. Two women developed their first symptoms during pregnancy, another patient noted a decrease of symptoms after the birth of her first child.

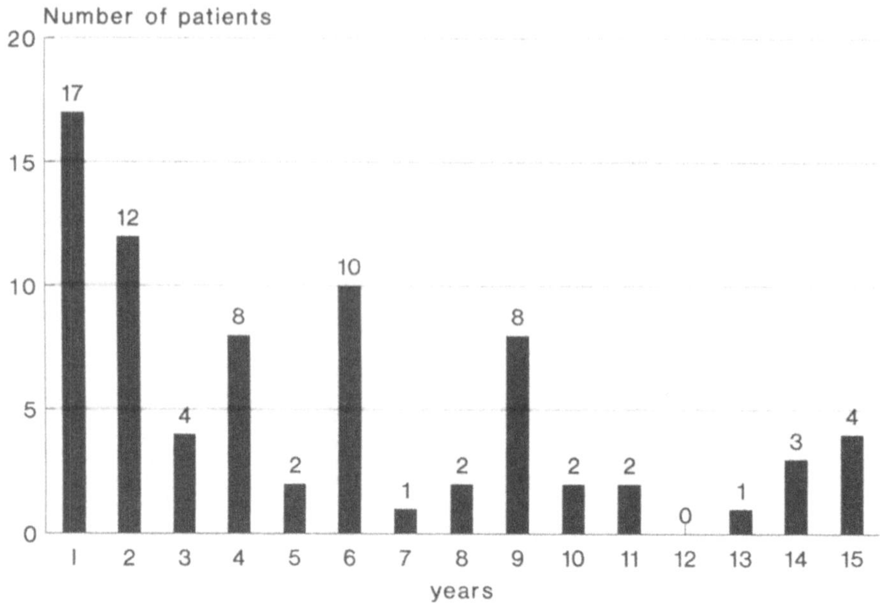

Fig. 2. Symptom-free interval after the first operation for Crohn's disease (mean 5.1 years; range 0–15 years)

In 32% of our patients an appendectomy was performed before the diagnosis of Crohn's disease. None of the appendectomies was incidental. The diagnosis of Crohn's disease became obvious in eight of the 34 appendectomy patients after histological examination of the appendix. In five other cases the histology of the appendix suggested Crohn's disease.

Thirty patients suffered initially from intestinal symptoms alone; eleven patients noted only extraintestinal symptoms. Initial abdominal pain was seen in 62% and diarrhoea in 57% of patients. Anal blood loss as an early symptom was diagnosed in 21% of patients, anal fistulae occurred at this stage in 13% of patients and intestinal fistulae were seen in 4% of patients.

The initial loss of weight was less than 5 kg in 15% of patients, between 5 and 10 kg in 24% and more than 10 kg in 21%. As an early symptom fever occurred in 24% of patients, stomatitis aphthosa only twice, and arthritis and erythema nodosum only once.

During the follow-up period the following complications of Crohn's disease were observed: in 43% of patients severe fistulae and/or abscesses and in 29% intestinal obstruction. Polyarthritis was diagnosed in 17% of patients and a cholecystolithiasis was demonstrated by ultrasonography or intraoperatively in 13% of patients. Additional findings in the follow-up period were nephrolithiasis in 11%, anal fissures in 10% and stomatitis aphthosa in 9% of patients. Less common were intestinal perforations into the peritoneal cavity, osteoporosis, anal blood loss and a stenosis of the ureter on the right side. In one 81-year-old lady a Duke's grade D adenocarcinoma of the descending colon was found. No other cancers were found.

Concerning aetiology only two patients had a history of medication with hydroxyquinoline. In one of these patients, Mexaform was prescribed in childhood for several months; the first symptom of Crohn's disease was diagnosed in this patient at the age of 20 years.

Of the 108 evaluated patients, 99 underwent a total of 252 operations (2.3 per patient, range 1–14). A total of 173 bowel resections were performed; in 33 cases an operation due of a fistula was performed at the same time. Fifty-one patients underwent surgery because of fistulae alone, nine patients never underwent an operation and 41 patients had only one operation. Twenty-one operations were performed because of recurrence in the region of a former anastomosis.

The mean interval from the first operation to a new manifestation of Crohn's disease was 5.1 years (range 0–15 years) (Fig. 2). In 51% of these patients the new manifestation occurred within 2 years of the operation.

Our patients were asked to classify their condition in comparison with the preoperative status as "better", "the same" or "worse". Seventy-eight per cent felt better, 14% the same and only 8% felt worse than before the first operation.

In this young population of patients with a mean age of 32 years at the start of disease, it is remarkable that 12% of patients are not able to do regular work at all and 28% can only work part-time; only 60% are in full-time employment.

Discussion

Compared with reports from the literature we could demonstrate only one single peak of age for the onset of the disease at between 20 and 25 years [1, 2, 6]. In spite of better knowledge and better diagnostic facilities the interval from first symptoms to diagnosis has in the last 55 years, since the first description of Crohn's disease, been reduced only from 4 to 3 years [1]; in our series it was reduced to a mean of 3.2 years. In the literature the rate of appendectomies before diagnosis is usually indicated as high, without exact figures being given [5, 7]. We found that 32% of our Crohn's disease patients had the condition after appendectomy. We also confirmed a high incidence of nephrolithiasis, which has also been reported previously [5].

On the other hand we could not confirm a second peak of high morbidity around 60 years of age as previously reported [2, 3]. Our female to male ratio was lower than described in the literature [1, 3–5]. A reduced fertility was not obvious in our group of patients [8]. Cholelithiasis occurred in 13% of patients, which is less than that found in similar studies. It was not possible to identify any drug or dietary influences related to the onset of Crohn's disease.

An increased rate of carcinoma was not found, a fact that may be due to the surgical approach of radical resection within healthy tissue. Increased rates of carcinomas are only described in series where bypass operations were the rule [9]. This may also apply in the case of stricturoplasty, but it is still too early to make a judgement based on follow-up results of this operation.

Although our patients represent a selected group of surgical Crohn's disease patients in a Central University Hospital in Switzerland, our data confirmed the principle findings reported by others in Switzerland and Central Europe [1–8]. The differences concerning lower incidence of cholelithiasis and the missing second peak of age around 60 years are noteworthy.

References

1. Fielding JF (1986) Clinical features of Crohn's disease in Ireland. Am J Gastroenterol 81: 524–528
2. Mekhjian HS, Switz DM, Melnyk CS, Rankin GB, Brooks RK (1979) Clinical features and natural history of Crohn's disease. Gastroenterology 77: 898–906
3. Fahrländer H, Shalev E (1974) Die Enterocolitis regionalis Crohn. Eine Verlaufs- und Vergleichsstudie anhand von 182 Patienten. Dtsch Med Wochenschr 99: 2207–2214
4. Fahrländer H, Baerlocher C (1971) Clinical features and epidemiological data on Crohn's disease in the Basle Area. Scand J Gastroenterol 6: 657–662
5. Tytgat G (1984) Morbus Crohn. In: Demling L (ed) Klinische Gastroenterologie, 2nd edn. Thieme, Stuttgart, pp 600–623
6. Goebell H, Förster S, Dirks E, Hotz J, Schaarschmidt K, Eigler FW (1987) Morbus Crohn: Klinische Erkrankungsmuster in Beziehung zur Lokalisation. Eine prospektive Analyse an 300 Patienten. Med Klin 82: 1–8
7. Hoffmann R, Maier KP (1988) Morbus Crohn des Dünndarmes. Pathologische, klinische und therapeutische Aspekte. Schweiz Rundschau Med Prax 77: 306–312
8. Mörl M, Rottler H, Hartwich G (1977) Schwangerschaftsverlauf bei Colitis ulcerosa und Morbus Crohn. Dtsch Med Wochenschr 102: 387–391
9. Glotzer DJ (1985) The risk of cancer in Crohn's disease. Gastroenterology 89: 438–441

Complications of Perianal Fistulae and Abscesses in Crohn's Disease: Detection by Fistulography Followed by Computed Tomography

L. Chapuis, D. Fournier, J.-C. Givel and P. Schnyder

Introduction

Crohn's disease is a chronic granulomatous inflammation which progresses from localized mucosal and submucosal lesions to extensive abscesses and fistulae, which are its most debilitating complications. They occur in at least 50% of all cases [3], and can involve all organs and structures adjacent to the diseased bowel.

Perirectal disease is very common in patients with Crohn's disease, and affects 75% of all patients with colitis and 25% of patients with small-bowel disease [6]. Perirectal abscesses and fistulae are often extensive because of a relative pain insensitivity peculiar to Crohn's disease. This leads to an advanced presentation which often makes effective treatment difficult. A defunctioning colostomy may be required, although this is seldom reversible with a satisfying clinical outcome [2].

A study of 21 patients followed for 10 years suggests that about a third of the fistulae heal spontaneously and a third heal after surgery, while a third of the patients will present with new fistulae after surgery [1].

Surgical drainage of acute perianal abscesses is always indicated for pain relief. This creates a fistula between the origin of the abscess and the perianal skin. Curative surgery is done electively when the intestinal disease, and especially proctitis, is quiescent because although surgery seldom exacerbates Crohn's disease, its results are much poorer if active disease is present.

This background of frequent spontaneous healing and the potential complications of early surgery suggest two roles for radiology in perianal Crohn's disease. All fistulae, abscesses and their local complications must be delineated precisely for optimal surgical treatment. Distant foci of active disease must also be sought to help in planning the appropriate timing for elective surgery. Single and double contrast barium enema and upper gastrointestinal studies with small-bowel follow-through are the classical radiological studies used for detecting mucosal abnormalities, enteroenteric fistulae and strictures [5]. However, computed tomography (CT) is superior for the detection and delineation of parietal and extraintestinal disease extension. In acute anorectal lesions, CT is the choice examination because it locates abscesses and other complications with precision. It is less invasive than contrast enema, especially when the patient is in severe pain. CT also has a much better contrast sensitivity than conventional radiography, allowing the demonstration of very small amounts of contrast media.

For these reasons, we felt that a combination of fistulography, with or without contrast enema, followed immediately by pelvic CT would be a very useful imaging procedure in long-standing cases of complicated perianal fistulae and abscesses where clinical examination is often difficult and sometimes misleading.

Patients

Only those patients who had long-standing fistulae which were resistant to conservative treatment, where distant complications were suspected, or where clinical examination was too painful to be satisfactory were studied. They were evaluated clinically by a surgeon experienced in anorectal diseases (JCG) before referral for radiologic examination.

Technique

We used a rounded needle, a soft rubber or Foley catheter to instill iodinated contrast in the fistulae. If the patient had more than one fistula, we used a water-soluble contrast enema because some vessels have a proximal valve-like mechanism which allows only antegrade filling.

Non-ionic contrast was used for fistulography because it is less painful in recently drained abscesses. The contrast was diluted for both fistulography and enema, since too high a concentration of iodine might cause artefacts on CT sections.

CT was then performed after taping small pieces of plastic over the fistulous openings and separating the buttocks with a small cotton wad. Initially we used contiguous 8-mm-thick sections, but we have recently discovered that thin-section high-resolution imaging using 4-mm slices every 6 mm gives a much better delineation of perirectal disease.

Fistulography was well tolerated, and no patient reported pain on injection of the contrast. This was probably due to the use of non-ionic contrast, and maybe also to the higher pain threshold of Crohn's disease patients. CT examination of the pelvis was fast, lasting at most 15 min, and was easy to perform. The images were of high quality with few motion artefacts in the pelvis.

Radiologic Results

Fistulography

Fistulography depicted sinus tracts, abscess cavities and communications between the bowel lumen and abscesses. This procedure did not, however, give a precise indication of the extension of fistulae and abscesses into soft tissue structures. It was, nevertheless, helpful in providing an overview of fistulae and abscess extension.

Computed Tomography

CT demonstrated numerous signs of Crohn's disease:

- Mucosal and parietal thickening, which is pathologic when the rectal wall exceeds 5 mm
- Perirectal fat thickening, with irregular streaks and numerous small lymph nodes, indicative of active disease [4]
- Blurring and disappearance of the fatty space between rectum wall and levator ani muscle, a good indication of inflammation extending beyond the bowel
- Abscess as a low-density cavity surrounded by an irregular dense capsule
- Osteomyelitis, with irregular bone destruction and sclerosis, and thickening and densification of the adjacent soft tissues [7]
- Fistulae rendered opaque by contrast, presenting as serpiginous tracts surrounded by dense, inflammatory tissue.

Cases

Case 1. A 46-year-old man with long-standing Crohn's disease had a perianal fistula for 2 years, which persistently drained purulent material. Fistulography showed a broad sinus tract extending from the rectum to the left buttock; the bowel lumen was opacified from the fistula. CT demonstrated precisely the point of passage of the fistula through the levator ani muscle, and also disclosed a small enterorectal fistula not known before (Fig. 1).

Case 2. A 21-year-old woman who had had untreated Crohn's disease for 3 years presented with an acute left para-anal abscess. When the abscess had been drained, fistulography did not disclose the sinus tracts; they were, however, demonstrated by CT as long submucosal fistulae owing to the superior contrast resolution of this technique (Fig. 2).

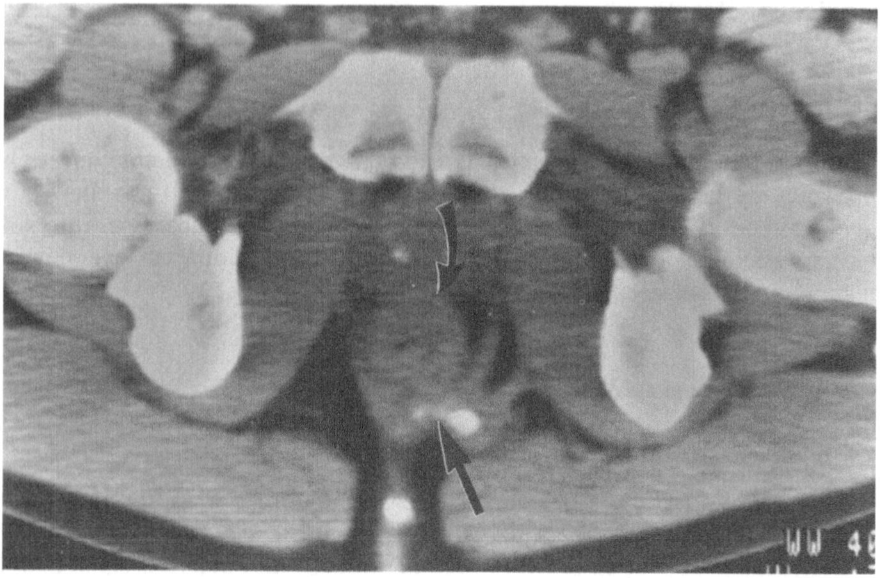

Fig. 1. Well-opacified fistula (*Straight arrow*) crossing the levator ani muscle. Moderate thickening of the bowel wall (*Curved arrow*)

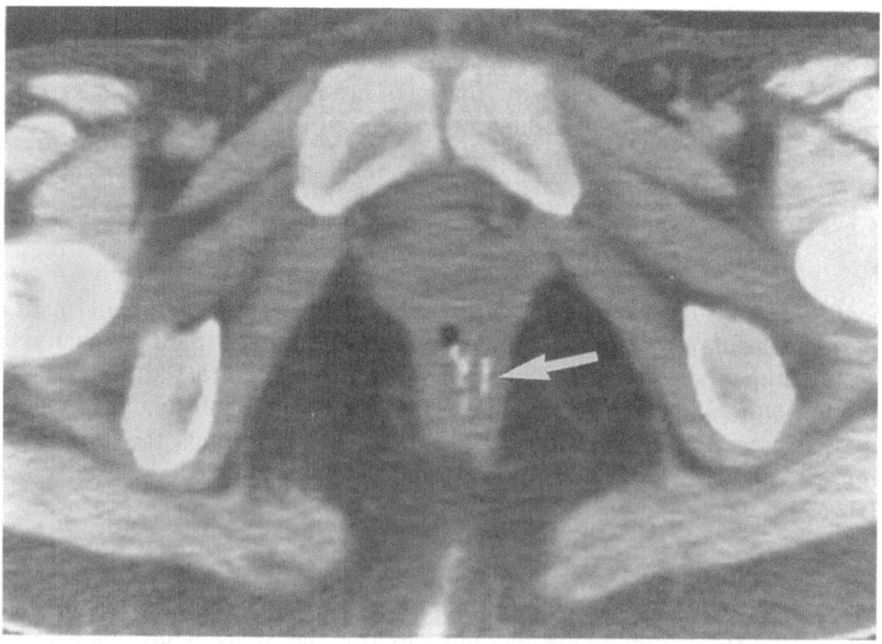

Fig. 2. Numerous thin parietal and perirectal fistulae (*arrow*). Complete loss of the normal fat space between levator ani and rectal wall, indicating severe inflammation

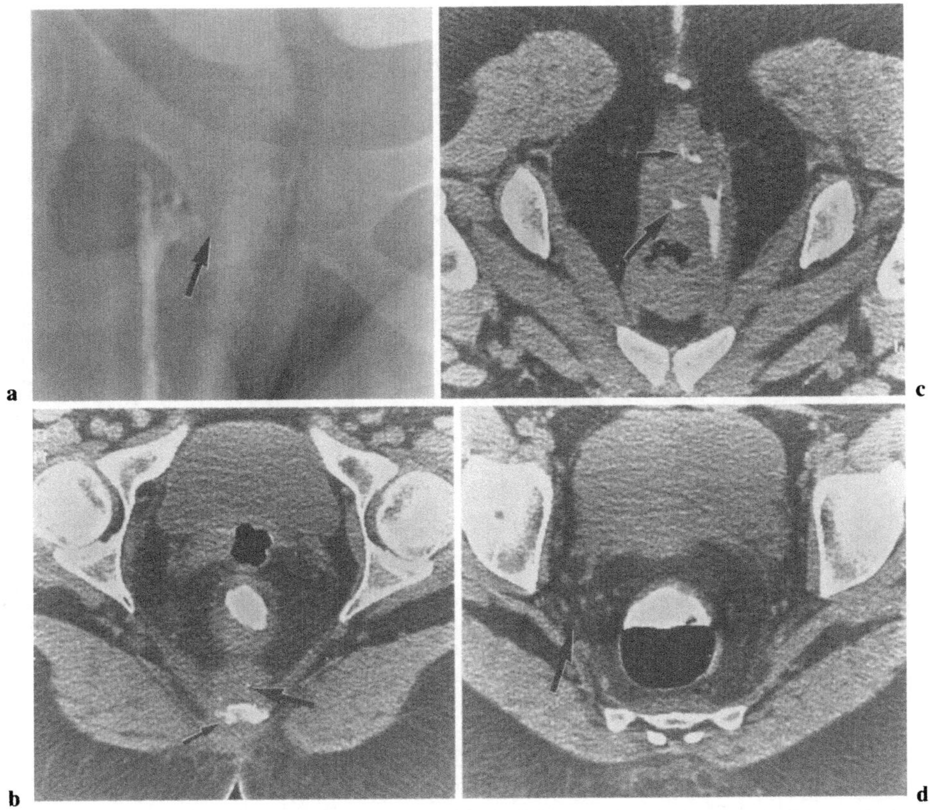

Fig. 3. **a** Fistulography shows a gas-containing abscess, with fistula to the rectal lumen (*arrow*). **b** Lower pelvic CT section demonstrating the abscess previously shown by fistulography and a second cavity (*small arrow*) behind the rectum (*large arrow*). Extensive inflammation of bowel wall and perirectal fat, with loss of the levator ani–rectum fat plane. **c** Marked rectal wall thickening. Presacral abscess partially opacified by contrast (*large arrow*), with bone erosion (*small arrow*) and soft tissue density very suggestive of osteomyelitis. **d** Numerous small lymph nodes (*arrow*) in the perirectal fat, indicative of chronic inflammation

Case 3. A 30-year-old woman with chronic Crohn's disease had an extensive perirectal abscess, which drained to the left buttock. Fistulography showed an abscess cavity and communication with the rectal lumen. However, CT demonstrated multiple cavities, a presacral abscess with suspected osteomyelitis, extensive thickening of the rectal mucosa, and disappearance of the usual fatty space between the levator ani muscle and the rectal wall (Fig. 3).

Case 4. A 53-year-old man had long-standing perianal abscesses and fistulae of unknown a etiology, the extent of which was well demonstrated by

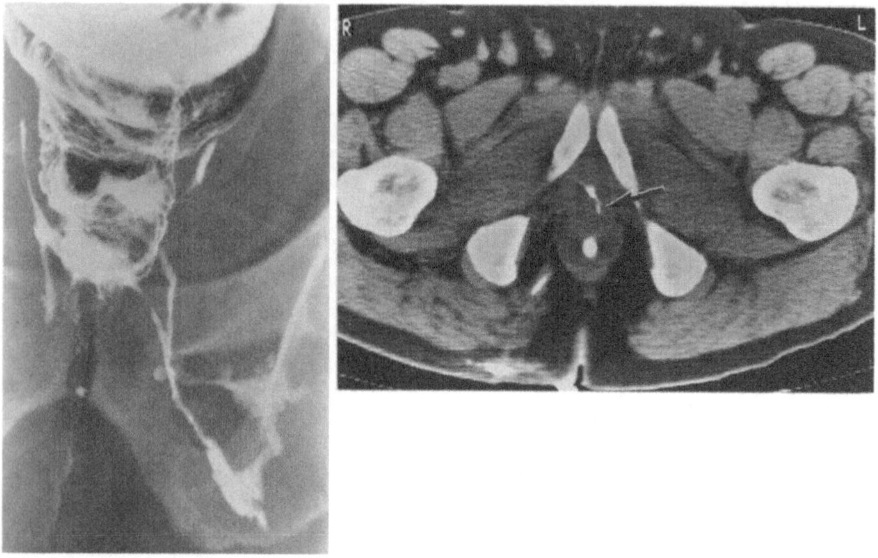

a b

Fig. 4. a Fistulography shows extensive perirectal fistulae and buttock abscesses. **b** CT section demonstrating two fistulous tracts, rectal thickening, and a recto-urinary fistula (*arrow*) with contrast meduim in the urethra

fistulography and contrast enema. However, CT disclosed the presence of a recto-urethral fistula not previously suspected (Fig. 4).

Conclusions

This report is a preliminary study evaluating the usefulness of CT combined with fistulography in the assessment of complex cases of perirectal fistulae and abscesses. Despite the limited number of patients examined to date due to the relative rarity of such extensive disease, we feel that some conclusions can already be drawn:

- CT disclosed previously unknown or unsuspected lesions in every case, and substantially improved upon the diagnostic accuracy of the fistulography.
- Fistulography is useful for a general survey of disease extension, but its use is very limited in the assessment of soft tissue and bone lesions.
- Clinical assessment in long-standing cases of perianal and perirectal fistulae is often difficult due to pain, fibrosis and scarring.

It remains to be seen whether this detailed evaluation has any impact on the clinical management, and ultimately on the outcome of these patients.

References

1. Buchmann P, Keighley MR, Allan RN, Thompson H, Alexander-Williams J (1980) Natural history of perianal Crohn's disease. Ten year follow-up: a plea for conservatism. Am J Surg 140: 642–644
2. Buchmann P, Weterman IT (1981) Der perianale Morbus Crohn. Colo-Proctology 3: 77–81
3. Donaldson RM (1989) Crohn's disease of the small bowel. In: Sleisenger MH, Fordtran JS (eds) Gastrointestinal disease, 4th edn. Saunders, Philadelphia, pp 1327–1358
4. Frager DH, Goldman M, Beneventano TC (1983) Computed tomography in Crohn's disease. J Comput Assist Tomogr 7: 819–824
5. Greenstein Orel S, Rubesin SE, Jones B, Fishman EK, Bayless TM, Siegelman SS (1987) Computed tomography vs barium studies in the acutely symptomatic patient with Crohn disease. J Comput Assist Tomogr 11: 1009–1016
6. Kelvin FM, Gedgaudas RK (1981) Radiologic diagnosis of Crohn disease (with emphasis on its early manifestations). Crit Rev Diagn Imaging 16: 43–91
7. Miller LK, Miller JW (1987) Pelvic osteomyelitis complicating Crohn's disease: diagnosis by Computed Tomography. Am J Gastroenterol 82: 371–373

Part IV: Complications

Ischaemic Lesions of the Intestine Due to Trauma

H. THOMPSON and T. MUSCROFT

Introduction

The development of abdominal symptoms or signs following assault, trauma or major surgery should alert the surgeon or clinician to the possibility of an ischaemic lesion of the intestines. If suspicion arises, laparotomy should be undertaken as an emergency since there is a risk of fatal perforation peritonitis. The occurrence of ischaemic colitis following major surgical operations due to hypovolaemia or to occlusion of the mesenteric arteries in aortic graft surgery is already well documented [1, 3, 4], but the risk following assault or accidental trauma is less well known [2, 5]. We describe a series of six cases which have come to our attention over the last 20 years.

Case 1

A 35-year-old man was admitted early on Christmas morning about 15 min after being stabbed in both arms whilst fending off an attack. On arrival at the hospital he was severely shocked, blood pressure was unrecordable and his pupils were dilated and unreactive to light. He was bleeding profusely from the wounds in both arms.

He was resuscitated with four units of 0-negative blood and 2.5 l of plasma. He regained consciousness with a systolic blood pressure of 80 mmHg. The wounds were immediately explored. In the right arm, the ulnar artery had been severed just distal to its origin. This was ligated. In the left arm there were two lacerations involving the triceps. Haemostasis was obtained, and the wounds were sutured. A further four units of blood were given during the operation.

Post-operatively the patient's progress was satisfactory. However, 19 h after the injury he complained of generalised abdominal pain and vomiting associated with a slightly distended abdomen but there were no localising signs and bowel sounds were present. He passed a quantity of altered blood with his stool. His vomit was streaked with blood 33 h after injury; the abdomen was more distended and tense, and there was tenderness and guarding in the right iliac fossa. Rectal examination revealed altered blood. Bowel sounds were now absent, the pulse was 100 beats per min and blood pressure was 140/100. The patient and witnesses of the assault denied any abdominal injury and no local bruising was evident on examination.

Laparotomy revealed gangrenous changes in the caecum, ascending colon and proximal transverse colon, and right hemicolectomy was performed. Post-operatively the patient made a good recovery and was discharged 14 days later with normal bowel function.

Case 2

A 22-year-old man was brought to the casualty department after cutting his right arm just below the axilla on a broken plate glass window. When first seen he was pulseless and nearly exsanguinated. Rapid infusion of plasma substitute and whole blood restored his blood pressure and he regained consciousness. Rapid bleeding recurred requiring firm digital pressure for control.

At immediate operation the brachial artery was found to be completely divided at its junction with the axillary artery, the major branches of the brachial plexus had been severed, and there was extensive muscle damage with bleeding. An end-to-end anastomosis of the artery restored the circulation of the limb. The nerves were marked to facilitate secondary repair.

The patient's immediate post-operative condition was satisfactory; he was conscious and alert with a good blood pressure and a satisfactory urinary output. He complained of vague abdominal pain, but there were no signs of peritonitis and bowel sounds were normal.

At this stage he had received ten units of blood, 2.2 l plasma substitute and two units of fresh frozen plasma, as well as crystalloid solutions. A further three units of whole blood were given later. The estimated interval between the occurrence of the injury and the restoration of a satisfactory blood pressure after controlling the artery was less than 60 min.

Some 20 h after the injury the patient complained of severe abdominal pain. On examination the abdomen was slightly distended and there was generalised tenderness and guarding. Laparotomy was carried out and the entire colon was found to be gangrenous down to the sigmoid colon and the mucosa was found to be necrotic as far distally as the mid rectum. Total colectomy and ileo-rectal anastomosis was performed.

Post-operatively, the patient developed septicaemic shock, which responded to antibiotics, methylprednisolone, and plasma infusion. Shortly thereafter a massive intra-abdominal haemorrhage led to his death.

Case 3

A boy, aged 8, fell off his bicycle. He sustained relatively minor head injuries with an orbital bruise and was detained in hospital for observation. Within 24 h he developed abdominal pain, vomiting, tachycardia, pyrexia of 102°F and abdominal tenderness. Laparotomy was undertaken which revealed an ischaemic lesion approximately 1½ in. in diameter in the sigmoid colon which was just beginning to leak (early perforation) with early peritonitis. Resection was carried out, and he made an uninterrupted recovery.

It was considered that the bicycle handlebars had caused a vascular injury (rupture, dissection or spasm) in a small artery in the mesentery of the sigmoid colon leading to ischaemic necrosis and imminent perforation.

Case 4

A 44-year-old man underwent a Whipple's resection for primary carcinoma of the duodenum. During mobilisation of the duodenum, a bleeding point was secured and a transitory bluish discolouration of the right side of the transverse colon was observed. Inspection of the bowel before closure showed normal colour and vascularity. The post-operative course was uneventful.

Three weeks later, the patient developed abdominal colic and vomiting which resolved. One week after this he had recurrent intestinal obstruction. Laparotomy revealed a firm stricture at the hepatic flexure. Resection was carried out and histology showed an ulcerated ischaemic stricture. A small artery which had been ligated and occluded was identified in the mesocolon.

Case 5

A man aged 27 was found unconscious after being involved in a fight. On recovery, he was groaning, holding his ribs and complaining of severe pain. There was a cut to his right ear and numerous abrasions and bruises. He was very drowsy and smelt strongly of alcohol. He was taken to hospital, examined and left to recover since there appeared to be no serious injuries. Several hours later he walked out of the casualty department and was taken to the police station. He vomited some blood and was taken back to hospital. There were no further developments and he was clinically stable. He was prescribed metoclopramide to avoid further vomiting and allowed to go home in a police car. During the journey he was holding his stomach and seemed to be in some discomfort. Next evening he deteriorated and was sent into hospital by the general practitioner. On admission there was abdominal tenderness and rigidity indicating perforation, and he was prepared for surgery. Fatal cardiac arrest occurred during induction of anaesthesia.

Autopsy revealed a small tear in the mesentery of the small intestine associated with an ischaemic lesion in the small bowel which had perforated leading to early peritonitis.

Case 6

A male lorry driver aged 36 was admitted to hospital as an emergency following a road traffic accident with a large perineal wound involving anus and rectum, avulsion of a piece of bone from ischial tuberosity and laceration of the left calf. A colostomy was introduced, and surgical repair of the perineal wound and débridement of the left calf was carried out. Skin graft procedures followed. The patient developed abdominal pain in the left iliac fossa and two faecal fistulae were present in the laparotomy wound 5 weeks later. He was admitted as an emergency 4 months later with a history of vomiting over the previous 2 weeks. The abdominal signs suggested obstruction. Laparotomy revealed cicatrising, necrotising colitis involving the entire colon accompanied by a perforation in the transverse colon. Purulent peritonitis was present and there was a large haematoma in the pelvis. Subtotal colectomy with ileostomy and sigmoidostomy was carried out. Fatal cardiac arrest occurred 6 days later. Histology showed cicatrising ischaemic colitis. There was no evidence of atheroma or cardiac disease at autopsy. The insurance company medical experts conceded that ischaemic colitis had been precipitated by the road traffic accident and substantial compensation was awarded to the patient's wife.

Discussion

Major trauma due to accident or assault and alcoholic intoxication may mask the development of ischaemic lesions of the intestine as a life-threatening complication. Surgical procedures and post-operative care directed towards the treatment of major injuries may overshadow an abdominal problem [2, 5]. Clinical symptoms and signs of an acute ischaemic lesion developed in four patients, and the other two presented weeks later with intestinal obstruction. Hypovolaemia and splanchnic vasoconstriction was an important factor in three cases (cases 1, 2 and 6). The hypovolaemic state was corrected by transfusion therapy fairly rapidly in all three patients, but nevertheless an ischaemic lesion developed. The protracted course of the intestinal lesion in case 6 is unusual, but this variety has been previously described as a chronic non-resolving form or as a subacute or chronic stricturing (mural form) of ischaemic colitis. Direct vascular injury accounted for the lesions in cases 3 and 4 and probably also in case 6. Surgical trauma with ligation of a small artery in the mesocolon led to an ischaemic stricture in the colon 4 weeks later in case 4. It is interesting that abdominal surgery had masked any acute signs which could have raised suspicions in the post-operative period; the first indication of the abdominal problem was consequently intestinal obstruction. Likewise the lesion in case 6 presented as an emergency with intestinal obstruction 4 months after injury although faecal fistula had been noted in the abdominal wound at a period of 5 weeks. In this case hypovolaemia, splanchnic vasoconstriction, vascular injury and possibly intestinal bacterial proliferation were involved in the mechanism and course of events. It is disappointing that the mortality rate in this small series was 50% despite surgical intervention.

References

1. Flynn TC, Rowlands BJ, Gilliland M, Ward RE, Fischer RP (1983) Hypotension-induced post-traumatic necrosis of the right colon. J Surg 146: 715–718
2. Guly HR, Steward IP (1982) Ischaemic colitis with perforation in a patient with multiple injuries. Injury 14: 100–102
3. Powis SJ, Barnes AD, Dawson-Edwards P, Thompson H (1972) Ileocolonic problems after cadaveric renal transplantation. BMJ 1: 99–101
4. Thompson H (1976) Ischaemic lesions of the intestines. Curr Views Gastroenterol 1: 153–170
5. Anonymous (1974) Seat belt injuries to the colon. BMJ 1:85–86

Management and Outcome of Diffuse Faecal and Purulent Peritonitis Due to Colonic Perforation

M. Gilg, W. Schweizer, G. Maddern, H.U. Baer, P. Gertsch and L.H. Blumgart

Introduction

The mortality in patients with diffuse and faecal peritonitis is reported to be between 15% and 40% [9, 10]. Because the number of such cases observed in a single institution is small, reports are usually carried out retrospectively over periods of up to 10 years [5]. It is therefore difficult to assess the progress made with recent improvements in antibiotic and intensive care treatment. Owing to the significant number of cases in our department we retrospectively reviewed the clinical records of patients who had presented with diffuse purulent or faecal peritonitis over the preceding 3 years.

Patients and Methods

In a retrospective study (1987–1989) 121 patients were reported to have a colonic perforation. In 28 of these patients a diffuse faecal or purulent peritonitis was found, which had extended to include more than two quadrants of the abdomen. We paid particular attention to the preoperative conditions of such patients, the time of treatment with antibiotics, the duration of hospitalisation, especially in an intensive care unit, and post-operative complications. Despite the relatively short follow-up period, all cases have been reviewed and their outcome following discharge had been established.

Results

Fifteen patients with a mean age of 71 years (range 42–84 years) had a diffuse purulent peritonitis and 13 patients with a mean age of 65 years (range 39–82 years) had a faecal peritonitis; 75% of the patients were over 60 years of age. There was an equal sex ratio. The mean interval between the onset of symptoms and admission was 5 days, with patients mainly

Table 1. Causes of colonic perforation

	Diffuse purulent peritonitis (*n*)	Diffuse faecal peritonitis (*n*)
Diverticular disease	13	4
Tumour perforation	2	6
Polyp resection	0	1
Colitis	0	2

complaining of nausea and abdominal discomfort followed by an acute onset of abdominal pain. Seventy per cent of our patients showed one or more risk factors at admission. Eleven patients were more than 20% overweight, seven patients had cardiac disease, three had pulmonary disease and two had renal disease. Two patients presented to our institution with a non-colonic carcinoma and one was human immunodeficiency virus (HIV) positive. Five patients had two or more risk factors. In all cases the diagnosis was made according to the clinical findings of peritonism from a plain abdominal X-ray which demonstrated free intraperitoneal air. All patients were operated on as emergencies. In 23 cases intraoperative bacteriology was performed, showing in 16 cases *Escherichia coli*, in six cases *Bacteroides*, in three cases *Pseudomonas*, *Klebsiella*, enterococcus and *Streptococcus* and in one case *Enterobacter*. The underlying disease was in 17 cases diverticulitis, in eight cases a tumour, in two cases a colitis and in one case a perforation following an endoscopic resection of a colonic polyp (Table 1).

On 22 occasions a Hartmann's procedure with the resection of the involved segment of the colon, closure of the rectal stump and terminal colostomy was performed after an extensive abdominal irrigation with several litres of saline solution. Two patients with acute colitis underwent a subtotal colectomy and terminal ileostomy, and in the one patient with an iatrogenic perforation the perforation was externalised with a loop transverse colostomy. One further case was intraoperatively misinterpreted as a perforation of acute appendicitis, and a caecostomy was performed, but postoperatively a histological finding of carcinoma in the appendix was made. On only one occasion was the perforation oversutured. There was one particularly desperate case in which only an explorative laparotomy was performed; this demonstrated an inoperable situation since there was no perfusion throughout the whole gut. No further surgical treatment was performed.

Postoperatively 40% of our patients needed intensive care unit management because of pulmonary dysfunction, or septic toxic shock for a mean period of 11 days (range 2–30 days). Two patients died within 24 h, a third patient died after 18 days. The remaining 25 patients survived and were discharged after a mean hospital stay of 29 days (range 11–75 days).

Table 2. Postoperative complications

	Diffuse purulent peritonitis		Faecal peritonitis	
	(*n*)	(%)	(*n*)	(%)
Death	1	7	2	15
Major wound dehiscence	1		4	
Minor wound dehiscence	4		2	
Cardiac insufficiency	1			
Renal insufficiency	1			
Necrotising fasciitis			1	
Haematoma			1	
Morbidity		52		75

Postoperatively 15 patients (60%) developed significant complications. On five occasions a further laparotomy was required because of a major wound dehiscence, and in a further six cases a minor wound dehiscence occurred. There was one case of severe cardiac insufficiency and one case of renal failure which required dialysis. One patient presented with necrotising fasciitis, in another a haematoma in the region of the rectal stump was found which required rectal drainage (Table 2).

All surviving patients were followed up until March 1990. In 11 the colostomy had been successfully closed. However, in one of these patients diffuse metastases were found during the procedure. Another patient died 7 months postoperatively because of overwhelming tumour growth. The remaining patients have not yet been reoperated on, although closure of the colostomy is envisaged in eight of them.

Discussion

Faecal and purulent peritonitis due to perforation of the colon still remains a serious disease. Such patients are usually elderly with serious concomitant diseases such as cardiac, respiratory or renal insufficiency. The presenting clinical picture usually takes some days to evolve and includes a slow deterioration in the patient's general condition. When they are seen in the hospital, patients are usually dehydrated and often in established septic shock. Such patients although in poor condition require urgent surgery. A mid-line laparotomy and careful exploration of the abdomen is the optimal approach. Broad spectrum antibiotic therapy should be started prior to anaesthesia and maintained for at least 5 days. We prefer to use penicillin, gentamycin and dalacin (clindamycin).

The operative strategy has been debated for many years, but the classical three-stage procedure of oversewing the perforation and protective colostomy, followed by resection of the colon as the second stage and closure of the colostomy as the third stage has today been abandoned [7]. The more recent approach has the advantage of a relatively short operating time for the severely ill patient who has diffuse peritonitis. However, due to improvements in anaesthetic care and resuscitation, a quick operation is no longer an essential consideration in deciding surgical management. When diverticular disease is the cause of the perforation the surgical procedure involves a sigmoid resection. In cases of perforation due to colonic cancer an adequate resection to gain tumour clearance must be conducted.

Recent reports have appeared suggesting that patients who undergo a direct anastomosis following colonic resection have a better prognosis than patients who undergo a two-stage or three-stage procedure [3, 11]. However, such an approach is only suitable for patients in relatively good physical condition. When the overall clinical situation is poor, the operative procedure performed is a Hartmann's procedure, for which a high mortality is reported [8–10]. Other authors recommend a laparotomy with daily repeat visits to the operating theatre for lavage and débridement [4]. The problem with this approach is that some of the patients require subsequent repair of a large ventral hernia which is not only technically difficult but has its own significant complications.

In our study we have been unable to demonstrate any significant differences in the outcome for patients suffering from either faecal or purulent peritonitis [6]. However, our numbers are small and a large series would be required to confirm this observation. Faecal peritonitis is more common in cases of colonic cancer and purulent peritonitis is often due to diverticular disease [5, 8]. It is often reported that a high mortality of between 50% and 70% occurs in cases of faecal peritonitis [1, 2]. This was not the finding in our group of patients. The complication rate is still a challenge for the future.

Conclusions

We found a relatively low mortality in patients with colonic perforation and diffuse peritonitis. The operative technique usually employed was a Hartmann's procedure, which was performed irrespective of the patient's general condition. Although the mortality was low, the morbidity remained high and patients had to undergo additional operations which necessitated a longer hospital stay. At the time of review 84% of the patients were alive.

References

1. Badia JM, Sitges-Serra A, Pla J, Ragné JM, Roqueta F, Sitges-Creus A (1987) Perforation of colonic neoplasms. A review of 36 cases. Int J Colorectal Dis 2: 187–189
2. Barth X, Fournier R, Padet JM, Vignal J, Lombard-Platet R (1988) Les perforations coliques en péritoine libre d'origine néoplasique. Choix thérapeutique. Chirurgie 114: 669–677
3. Cady J, Godfroy J, Sibaud O (1988) L'anastomose colo-rectale mécanique d'urgence en péritoine septique. A propos d'une série de quarante-six péritonites par perforation sigmoïdienne dont trente généralisées. Ann Chir 42: 647–651
4. Eigler FW, Coone HJ (1987) Kolonperforation. Dtsch Med Wochenschr 112: 144–147
5. Ellis H (1989) Perforated diverticulitis of the colon. Dig Surg 6: 162–164
6. Guyton DP, Evans D, Schreiber H (1985) Stercoral perforation of the colon. Concepts of operative management. Am Surg 51: 520–522
7. Hartmann H (1931) Nouveau procédé d'ablation des cancers de la partie terminale du côlon pelvien. Trentième congrès de chirurgie, Strasbourg, p 411
8. Khaergaard J, Fischer AB, Baden H (1984) Hartmann's operation as an emergency procedure for perforation of the sigmoid colon. A consecutive series. Acta Chir Scand 150: 255–257
9. Krukowski ZH, Matheson NA (1984) Emergency surgery for diverticular disease complicated by generalized and faecal peritonitis: a review. Br J Surg 71: 921–927
10. Nagorney DM, Adson MA, Pemberton JH (1985) Sigmoid diverticulitis with perforation and generalized peritonitis. Dis Colon Rectum 28: 71–75
11. Weddel J, Banzhaf G, Mrohs A, Fischer R (1989) Plädoyer für die primäre Resektion mit primärer Anastomose bei der komplizierten Sigmadivertikulitis. Erfahrungsbericht der Chirurgischen Klinik Herford 1973 bis 1986. Langenbecks Arch Chir 374: 259–266

Treatment of Colonic Anastomotic Strictures with "Through the Scope" Balloon Dilators

M.D. DINNEEN and R.W. MOTSON

Introduction

Anastomotic strictures occur in 1.2%–4.2% of all patients undergoing colonic resection [1]. They are reported to be more common with two-layer than with single-layer or stapled anastomoses [2]. Symptomatology correlates poorly with stricture diameter, and some strictures 1 cm in diameter may be completely asymptomatic [3].

Benign colonic anastomotic strictures may result from ischaemia, haemorrage or leakage at the suture line or from recurrent Crohn's disease. Inflammation and fibrosis develop as a consequence. There may be a prolonged active fibrotic process and it may be that early endoscopic intervention could break this cycle.

Some early anastomotic strictures seem to resolve spontaneously but for those that remain symptomatic or do not respond to conservative measures, re-resection or some other abdominal procedure may have to be considered. Balloon dilatation offers a less radical solution.

The first description of the clinically successful use of balloon dilatation catheters appeared in the German literature in 1974, when Gruntzig described balloon dilatation of atheromatous narrowings of the iliac, femoral and popliteal vessels [4]. The technique was first applied to the gastrointestinal tract in 1980 when London treated oesophageal strictures in this manner [5]. In 1983, Ball dilated ischaemic strictures of infant colons with balloon catheters, using a Seldinger technique under fluoroscopic control [6]. Brower and Freeman in 1984 described balloon dilatation of a large-bowel stricture in an adult [7].

Materials and Methods

The technique employed utilises microvasive Rigiflex® "through the scope" (TTS) balloon dilatation catheters. Following standard colonoscopic preparation the stricture is visualised and the balloon catheter is passed through the stricture. Colonic balloon dilatation catheters are available in four sizes (Fig. 1): 30, 36, 45 and 54 Fr gauge. The balloon length is 8 cm and the shaft length is 180 cm. The pressure required to inflate the balloon decreases as the diameter increases; the 30 Fr catheter requires 55 psi whereas the 54 Fr requires 35 psi. Once in position across the stricture the balloon is inflated with water for a period of 1 min. A brief description of the first three patients in whom we have performed this technique follows:

Patient 1. A 59-year-old male presented with an acute abdomen. At laparotomy he was found to have peritonitis, secondary to a perforated paracolic abscess. He underwent a Hartmann's procedure. Four months later this was reversed; the anastomosis was fashioned with vicryl in one layer. One month after this operation he presented with the symptoms and signs of subacute obstruction. Barium enema demonstrated an anastomotic stricture (Fig. 2). He underwent TTS balloon dilatation and this resulted in a complete resolution of his symptoms. Further endoscopy at 6 and 18 months was normal and the patient was discharged.

Patient 2. A 71-year-old female presented acutely with a large-bowel obstruction. An extensive rectal carcinoma was discovered. She underwent an anterior resection with on-the-table lavage and primary stapled anastomosis. She remained asymptomatic for 15 months and then presented again with large-bowel obstruction. At endoscopy she was found to have an anastomotic stricture at 10 cm; TTS balloon dilatation was performed immediately and her symptoms resolved. Two months later she again developed large-bowel obstruction as the stricture had recurred. Repeat TTS dilatation was performed and again her symptoms resolved completely. She remained asymptomatic until her death 4 months later from liver secondaries.

Patient 3. The third patient was a 29-year-old female who underwent a limited ileo-caecal resection and transverse colectomy for Crohn's disease. Both anastomoses were fashioned in one layer with Dexon. Two months post-operatively her symptoms recurred and barium studies demonstrated a tight colonic stricture and a less tight ileocolic stricture (Fig. 3). TTS balloon dilatation was carried out on the distal stricture. After this, however, it was not possible to advance the colonoscope through the stricture. There was only a minimal improvement in the patient's symptoms. Six months later repeat TTS dilatation was performed, this time on both strictures. The larger 75 Fr balloon dilatation was used. Shortly after the procedure the patient developed abdominal pain. On examination she was found to have peritonism and at laparotomy was discovered to have had a perforation at the site of the colonic stricture. A stricturoplasty was performed, and she is now asymptomatic 6 months later.

TTS balloon dilatation has now been successfully carried out on a further two patients with colonic anastomotic strictures although follow-up is only of short duration.

Discussion

In a national survey of endoscopists carried out in 1986 Kozarek collected information on 64 balloon dilatations of colonic strictures of varied aetiology. These were exclusively performed by the Seldinger technique predominantly under fluoroscopic control. Kozarek noted that when the balloon diameter was less than 40 Fr, less than 50% of the patients benefited. Increasing the balloon diameter to 51 Fr or greater led to over 90% symptomatic improvement [8]. In an earlier paper, the same author recommended that for an effective hydrostatic force to be generated pressures of the order of 20–60 psi should be maintained for periods of 15–60 s [9].

The advantages of this technique are numerous. It allows the endoscopist direct visualisation thereby maximising his control over the procedure. As the balloon is inflated radial pressures are generated, as opposed to the longitudinal and shearing forces of traditional bouginage. In theory this should decrease the risk of viscus perforation. The balloon itself is made of an inelastic polymer and can only be inflated to its designed maximum diameter. Excess pressure does not cause an increase in balloon diameter as would occur with a latex balloon. The procedure is minimally invasive and results in a much shorter hospital stay than operative resection of the stricture. Most importantly it appears to be an effective and relatively safe procedure, although is not without risk.

The complications of the technique are bowel perforation, as previously described. In Kozarek's series there were three perforations in 64 dilatations and two of these occurred at anastomotic strictures. Significant haemorragic complications were reported in two of the 64 cases [8]. Colonoscopic complications such as adverse drug reactions, aspiration and cardiorespiratory events must also be mentioned.

In conclusion, this is a preliminary report on a new technique. We believe that TTS balloon dilatation of colonic anastomotic strictures is an effective treatment which has a role to play in the treatment of patients with symptomatic strictures that would otherwise require resection.

References

1. Thies E, Lange V, Miersch WD (1983) Peranal dilatation of a postsurgical colonic stenosis by means of a flexible endoscope. Endoscopy 15: 327–328
2. Langer S (1978) Colon-Nahttechnik: Einreihige Naht. Langenbecks Arch Chir 347: 601–604
3. Mazier WP (1973) A technique for the management of low colonic anastomotic stricture. Dis Colon Rectum 16: 113–116
4. Grüntzig A, Hopff H (1974) Perkutane Rekanalisation chronischer arterieller Verschlüsse mit einem neuen Dilatationskatheter. Dtsch Med Wochenschr 99: 2502–2505

5. London RL, Trotman BW, DiMarino AJ, Oleaga JA, Freiman DB, Ring EJ, Rosato EF (1981) Dilatation of severe esophageal strictures by an inflatable balloon catheter. Gastroenterology 80: 173–175
6. Ball WS, Seigel RS, Goldthorn JF, Kosloske AM (1983) Colonic strictures in infants following intestinal ischemia. Radiology 149: 469–472
7. Brower RA, Freeman LD (1984) Balloon catheter dilation of a rectal stricture. Gastrointest Endosc 30: 95–97
8. Kozarek RA (1986) Hydrostatic balloon dilation of gastrointestinal stenoses: a national survey. Gastrointest Endosc 32: 15–19
9. Kozarek RA (1984) Endoscopic Gruntzig balloon dilation of gastrointestinal stenoses. J Clin Gastroenterol 6: 401–407

Clinical Assessment in Pouchitis: Is It Accurate in Diagnosis?

W.A. Kmiot and M.R.B. Keighley

Introduction

The pathogenesis of pouchitis is unknown [1]. Proposed aetiological factors have included faecal stasis and bacterial overgrowth [2], recurrent Crohn's disease [3], recurrent ulcerative colitis [4] and specific enteropathogens [5]. However, many of the cases of pouchitis described in the literature have not been fully documented using the now recognised clinical, endoscopic and histological criteria [4].

Pouchitis is a specific complication found in ileal reservoirs but the criteria used to diagnose pouchitis vary between different centres. Some centres use a combination of clinical, sigmoidoscopic and histological criteria [1, 2] whilst others use clinical and sigmoidoscopic criteria alone [6]. In one study the diagnosis of pouchitis in some patients was based on symptoms reported on the telephone [7]. It is not surprising therefore that the incidence of pouchitis is so variable: 44% [5], 7% [6], 22% [4] and 10% [1].

The aim of this study, therefore, is to establish whether clinical criteria alone can be used to predict the presence of acute inflammatory changes in the pouch mucosa. Furthermore, operative techniques have been studied to provide insight into their role in the aetiology of pouchitis.

Patients and Methods

The first 70 patients to have undergone ileal pouch-anal anastomosis in Birmingham were studied.

All 70 subjects were divided into four groups based on the four major changes in surgical technique observed during one surgeon's evolving experience. The four variables were: (a) extent of rectal resection and mucosal proctectomy, (b) use of selective vascular mobilisation, (c) pouch design and (d) technique of ileo-anal anastomosis.

Specific operative details for each group were recorded as was the incidence of post-operative pouch excision, pelvic sepsis, anal stricture and

Table 1. Sigmoidoscopic scoring system used to grade the severity of acute pouch inflammation

	Sigmoidoscopic aspect	Score
1	Loss of vascular pattern	1
2	Mucosal granularity	2
3	Contact haemorrhage	3
4	Spontaneous haemorrhage	4
5	Mucosal ulceration	5
6	Surface mucopus	6

per-operative steroid therapy. The association of these factors with pouchitis was investigated using prospectively collated patient records.

Functional results for patients with an intact ileal reservoir were detailed during a personal interview at which each subject completed a written questionnaire relating to pouch function at 3, 6, 12, 24 and 36 months following ileostomy closure.

Frequency of defaecation by day and by night was recorded as was the need for anti-diarrhoeal medication. Soiling was defined as faecal leakage through the anus sufficient to require use of a pad more than once a week. Urgency was assessed by asking the patient how long defaecation could be deferred after the first call to stool. Urgency was classified as severe if defaecation could not be deferred for 10 min, whilst moderate urgency was defined as a maximum time to defer defaecation of 10–30 min. Episodes of incontinence to liquids and semi-solids were recorded. Adequate discrimination between flatus and faeces was judged to be present if the patients could pass wind safely without visiting the toilet.

Following clinical assessment all patients underwent sigmoidoscopy on the same day. Sigmoidoscopic results were graded using previously defined criteria of acute inflammation [1] (Table 1). As pouchitis has a patchy distribution, the highest grade of inflammation was recorded to facilitate standardisation. Patient scores were determined by a single person who had not been involved in operative management. All patients with pouch inflammation of macroscopic grade greater than or equal to 3 underwent biopsy from an inflamed area in order to exclude Crohn's disease. A single random stool was also collected from each patient with pouchitis and cultured for *Salmonella*, *Shigella*, *Campylobacter*, *Clostridium difficile* bacterium and toxin as well as for ova, cysts and parasites.

To avoid the assumption of a normal distribution the data is expressed as the median and 95% confidence intervals. Independent values in two unpaired groups were analysed using the Wilcoxon text. Unpaired groups of more than two in number were analysed using a one-way rank analysis of variance. Paired data for two groups were analysed using the Wilcoxon signed rank test. For paired groups of more than two in number a two-way rank analysis of variance was employed.

Table 2. Patient stratification into the four study groups

	Patient groups			
	First 18 pouches[a]	Next 16 J pouches	16 W pouches	20 J pouches
Age (median, range)	30(20–42)	33(27–43)	37(24–42)	30(20–41)
Sex				
Female	11	8	8	13
Male	7	8	8	7
Diagnosis				
UC	17	11	13	14
FAP	0	2	1	3
Constipation	1	3	2	3

Data are given as the median and 95% confidence intervals. UC, ulcerative colitis; FAP, familial adenomatous polyposis
[a] 2 S and 16 J pouches

Correlations were made using Spearman's rank test and proportions were analysed using a Fisher exact test. Significance was assumed if $p < 0.05$ using a two-tailed test.

Results

The 70 patients in the study divided into four chronological groups:

1. The first 18 pouches (2 S and 16 J)
2. The next 16 J pouches
3. The first 16 W pouches
4. The first 20 totally stapled J pouches

Patients

There was no significant difference between the median and 95% confidence intervals of the four sequential patient groups with respect to age ($p = 0.65$), sex distribution (significance range $p = 0.57$–0.99) and proportion of patients with a diagnosis of ulcerative colitis (significance range $p = 0.12$–0.92) (Table 2).

Further details of differences between the four groups regarding previous colectomy, covering ileostomy, method of pouch formation and ileo-anal anastomosis, extent of mucosal protectomy and length of rectal cuff, preservation of anal transition zone and extent of vascular division are given in Table 3.

Table 3. Variability in operative techniques used in the four study groups

	First 18 pouches	Next 16 J pouches	16 W pouches	20 J pouches
Previous colectomy	13	9	11	6
Covering ileostomy	15	11	10	5
Pouch construction				
Sutured	9	0	16	0
Stapled	9	16	0	20
Ileo-anal anastomosis				
Sutured	18	16	16	0
Stapled	0	0	0	20
Mucosal proctectomy				
Endoanal	9	0	0	0
Abdominal	9	16	16	0
Rectal cuff				
Long	9	0	0	0
Short	9	16	16	20
Anal transition zone				
Preserved	0	3	3	20
Excised	18	13	13	0
Vascular division				
Minimal	18	0	0	20
Extensive	0	16	16	0

Table 4. Details of post-operative complications

	First 18 pouches	Next 16 J pouches	16 W pouches	20 J pouches
Pouch excision				
Early	0	1	1	1
Late	7	1	0	0
Pelvic sepsis				
Total (laparotomy)	9(9)	2(2)	2(1)	5(4)
Fistula	6	0	2	1
Ileo-anal leak	9	2	2	4
Anal stenosis (intubation)	5(1)	2(0)	2(0)	2(0)
Per-operative steroids	3	0	0	3
Pouchitis	4	4	4	4

Post-Operative Complications (*Table 4*)

Over 60% of all pouch excisions occurred in the first 18 patients (7/18); this compares with two excisions in the sutured J pouches (2/16; $p = 0.17$), one in the group of 16 W pouches (1/16; $p = 0.06$) and one in the 20 totally stapled J pouch group (1/20; $p = 0.028$). The only patient in whom excision was required for pouchitis had an extensive vascular mobilisation at the time of ileal pouch formation and an anal stricture.

There was no statistically significant difference in the incidence of pelvic sepsis between the four study groups despite the number being higher in the first 18 pouches (9/18) compared with the other groups (next 16 J pouches, 2 out of 16, $p = 0.09$; the 16 W pouches, 2 out of 16, $p = 0.09$ and the totally stapled J pouch group, 5 out of 20, $p = 0.36$. The incidence of pelvic sepsis was unrelated to either length of rectal cuff and method of mucosectomy (long cuff and endoanal mucosectomy $n = 5$, short cuff and abdominal mucosectomy $n = 4$) or to previous colectomy (with colectomy $n = 9$, without colectomy $n = 9$).

Twelve patients developed an anal stricture, four of whom had a previous episode of pelvic sepsis. However, there was no significant difference in the incidence of anal stricture between the four study groups (first 18, 5/18; next 16 J, 2/16; 16 W, 2/16 and 20 stapled J, 3/20). Although all six patients on per-operative steroid therapy at the time of ileal pouch formation developed pelvic sepsis, none of them later developed pouchitis.

Pouchitis

Sixteen patients (23%) have developed pouchitis after restorative proctocolectomy. Four out of the 16 patients with pouchitis had an anal stricture. A further four patients with pouchitis but without anal strictures had a history of pelvic sepsis. Equal numbers of patients in this series had pouchitis irrespective of whether an extensive vascular mobilisation had been ($n = 8$) or had not been ($n = 8$) performed at the time of ileal reservoir formation. Neither pouch design (J, 4/16; W, 4/16), nor method of ileo-anal anastomosis (sutured J, 4/16; stapled J, 4/20) was associated with the development of pouchitis. No patient with pouchitis was later found to have Crohn's disease. Faecal bacterial culture failed to reveal any specific enteropathogens in patients with pouchitis.

Fifteen of the 16 patients with pouchitis had ulcerative colitis and one patient had familial adenomatous polyposis. The extent of ulcerative colitis in the colectomy specimens from these 15 patients was total in 14 out of 15 patients and distal in the remaining patient. The first attack of pouchitis varied from 3 months to 36 months following ileal pouch construction. Pouchitis was not found in any patient following ileal pouch formation for constipation. None of the pouchitis patients had any evidence of backwash ileitis in their colectomy specimens.

Only three patients had recurrent episodes of pouchitis following initial treatment with metronidazole. All recurrent episodes of pouchitis responded to further metronidazole except in one patient for whom steroid enemas and sulphasalazine therapy was necessary.

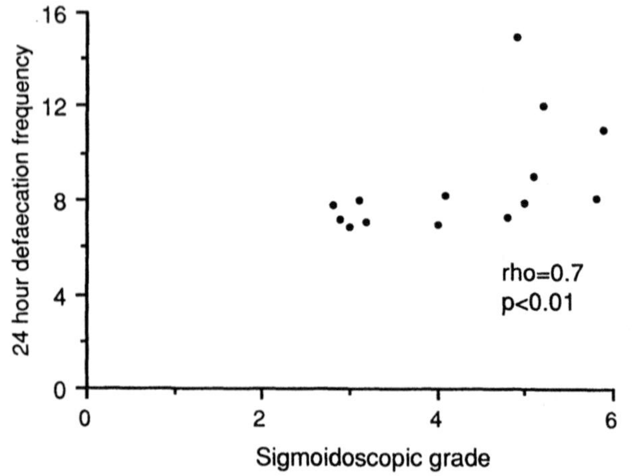

Fig. 1. Correlation of sigmoidoscopic grade of acute pouch inflammation with urgency grade

Functional Result

Patients were only assessed for functional result if their ileostomy had been closed for a minimum of 3 months. This left a total of 53 patients (first 18 pouches $n = 8$; next 16 J pouches $n = 14$; 16 W pouches $n = 15$; 20 stapled J pouches $n = 16$). Fourteen of these 53 patients had pouchitis. All comparisons of clinical and sigmoidoscopic criteria for patients with and without pouchitis were made at similar times following ileostomy closure.

All patients with a sigmoidoscopic grade of 3–6 were classified as having pouchitis, as this grade range has been previously shown to be associated with the histological features of pouchitis [1].

Pouchitis patients had either a moderate or severe degree of urgency. Severe urgency was seen only in patients with pouchitis ($n = 7$) but moderate urgency was present not only in pouchitis patients ($n = 7$) but also in patients without pouchitis ($n = 6$). Urgency therefore has a negative predictive value of 100% and a positive predictive value of 66% in the diagnosis of pouchitis. Furthermore, there was no correlation between urgency and sigmoidoscopic grade in pouchitis patients (Fig. 1).

All pouchitis patients soiled at night and five pouchitis patients also soiled during the day. However, 15 patients without pouchitis also soiled at night and five of these patients also soiled during the day. Thus nocturnal soiling has a negative predictive value of 100% and a positive predictive value of 44% in the diagnosis of pouchitis.

Twelve of the 14 pouchitis patients required anti-diarrhoeal medication and ten out of these 14 patients were able to discriminate flatus from faeces during an acute attack of pouchitis.

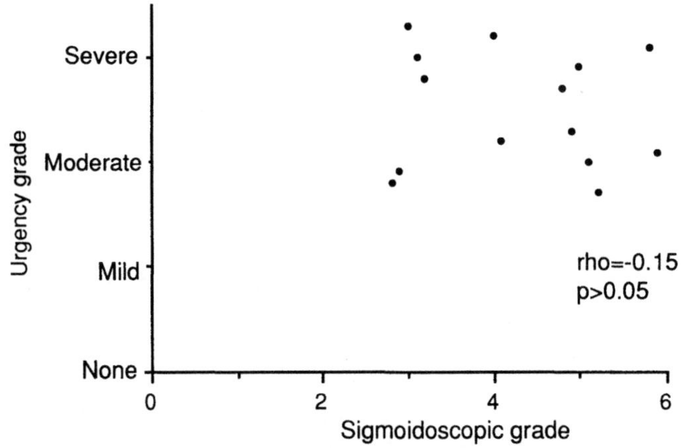

Fig. 2. Correlation of sigmoidoscopic grade of acute pouch inflammation with 24-h frequency of defaecation

Frequency of defaecation in a 24-h period was equal to or greater than seven times in all patients with pouchitis. However, 20 patients without pouchitis also had the same high frequency of defaecation over 24 h. Therefore frequency of defaecation of greater than or equal to seven over 24 h had a negative predictive value of 100% and a positive predictive value of 37% in the diagnosis of pouchitis. Nevertheless, there was a significant correlation between the frequency of defaecation over 24 h and sigmoidoscopic grade in pouchitis (Fig. 2).

Discussion

This study has shown that no specific operative factor in restorative proctocolectomy influences the development of pouchitis. In addition, none of the following factors were shown to be associated with pouchitis: pelvic sepsis, anal stricture or per-operative steroid therapy.

The overall rate of complications remained high throughout the series with only 20%–30% of patients within the four subgroups free of any complication, a situation similar to that described in the Mayo clinic [8].

A learning curve was demonstrated with over 60% of pouches that required excision occurring in the first 18 patients, although half of these patients required pouch excision for the sequelae of pelvic sepsis. However, the overall rate of pelvic sepsis of 26% in this series is similar to the 8%–22% recorded from a recent symposium [9], although the rate of anal stricture formation is higher in this study (17%).

Like others we have not shown that reservoir design is important in the aetiology of pouchitis [1]. A new finding, however, was that extensive vascular mobilisation, type of ileo-anal anastomosis and extent of mucosal proctectomy did not influence the incidence of pouchitis. The study also showed that pouchitis can occur independent of a previous diagnosis of ulcerative colitis [3] and without the colectomy specimen exhibiting total colitis [10].

As all pouchitis patients presented urgency, nocturnal soiling and a 24-h defaecation frequency equal to or greater than seven, the negative predictive values of these three parameters was 100%. The low positive predictive values of these three parameters, however, is not surprising as other factors including low pouch compliance [11], impaired anal sphincter function [12], motility disturbances of the small bowel [13] and jejunal bacterial overgrowth [2] may present with similar symptoms following restorative proctocolectomy.

Thus clinical assessment alone does not accurately diagnose pouchitis and a sigmoidoscopic assessment should always be made to confirm a clinical impression of pouchitis. Furthermore, the aetiology of pouchitis is unlikely to be related to specific mechanical aspects of ileal reservoir construction.

References

1. Moskowitz RL, Shepherd NA, Nicholls RJ (1986) An assessment of inflammation in the reservoir after restorative proctocolectomy with ileoanal ileal reservoir. Int J Colorectal Dis 1: 167–174
2. O'Connell PR, Rankin DR, Weiland LH, Kelly KA (1986) Enteric bacteriology, absorption, morphology and emptying after ileal pouchanal anastomosis. Br J Surg 73: 909–914
3. Tytgat GN, Van Deventer SJ (1988) Pouchitis. Int J Colorectal Dis 3: 226–228
4. Madden MV, Farthing MJ, Nicholls RJ (1990) Inflammation in ileal reservoirs: "pouchitis". Gut 31: 247–249
5. Fleshman JW, Cohen Z, McLeod RS, Stern H, Blair J (1988) The ileal reservoir and ileoanal anastomosis procedure. Factors affecting technical and functional outcome. Dis Colon Rectum 31: 10–16
6. Hulten L (1986) In: Symposium restorative proctocolectomy with ileal reservoir. Int J Colorectal Dis 1: 17
7. Goldberg SM, Rothenberger DA (1986) In: Symposium restorative proctocolectomy with ileal reservoir. Int J Colorectal Dis 1: 15–16
8. Pemberton JH, Kelly KA, Beart RW, Dozois RR, Wolff BG, Ilstrup DM (1987) Ileal pouch-anal anastomosis for chronic ulcerative colitis. Long-term results. Ann Surg 206: 504–513
9. Williams NS (1986) In: Symposium restorative proctocolectomy with ileal reservoir. Int J Colorectal Dis 1: 2–9
10. Farrands P, Nicholls RJ (1989) Paper presented to the Association of Surgeons of Great Britain and Ireland
11. Nasmyth DG, Johnston D, Godwin PG, Dixon MF, Smith A, Williams NS (1986) Factors influencing bowel function after ileal pouch-anal anastomosis. Br J Surg 73: 469–473

12. Nicholls RJ, Belliveau P, Neill M, Wilks M, Tabaqchali S (1981) Restorative proctocolectomy with ileal reservoir: a pathophysiological assessment. Gut 22: 462–468
13. Heppell J, Kelly KA, Phillips SF, Beart RW, Telander RL, Perrault J (1982) Physiologic aspects of continence after colectomy, mucosal proctectomy and endorectal ileo-anal anastomosis. Ann Surg 195: 435–443

Part V: Miscellaneous

Colonic Perforation in an Immunocompromised Host

M. Dusmet and G. Chapuis

Introduction

The spectrum of disease associated with human immunodeficiency virus (HIV) infection is considerable. The gastrointestinal tract is particularly prone to disease in these patients and both diarrhoea and weight loss are common symptoms; HIV itself has been implicated in their pathogenesis. Other common infecting agents include parasites (*Cryptosporidium*, *Isospora belli* and *Giardia lamblia*), bacteria (*Salmonella*, *Shigella*, etc.), atypical bacteria (*Mycobacterium avium intracellulare* complex, MIC) and viruses (notably cytomegalovirus, CMV, and other herpes viruses). Besides infective diarrhoea these patients can present with gastrointestinal haemorrhage, obstruction by or perforation from Kaposi's sarcoma, lymphoma or inflammatory diseases (which can cause both ulceration and a pseudo Crohn's disease). Furthermore, both CMV and *Cryptosporidium* can cause a specific form of hepatobiliary disease in these patients.

Case Report

The patient was a 30-year-old female with a past history of head trauma and epileptic seizures due to intermittent barbiturate withdrawal (she commonly abused "over-the-counter" painkillers containing barbiturates), who denied i.v. drug abuse. She was a social drop-out with no professional training and a possible past history of anorexia nervosa. In the summer of 1988, she was found to be HIV positive (from sexual contact with i.v. drug abusers). In early May 1989, she presented with severe watery, blood-stained diarrhoea. Rectosigmoidoscopy demonstrated diffuse inflammation and ulceration. Four biopsies were taken and considered to be compatible with ulcerative colitis. No pathogens or CMV inclusions were identified, although carefully sought.

She was admitted to our hospital in mid-May and a complete and extensive work-up again failed to identify any of the pathogens commonly associated with colitis in HIV-positive patients. With great hesitation prednisone (40 mg/day, then 20 mg/day) was introduced with no change in her clinical course. On June 20, she presented with sudden abdominal pain, guarding and free air on plain abdominal X-rays. A laparotomy was performed and two tiny perforations of the right and sigmoid colon were found and oversewn and covered with an omental patch. The abdomen was closed after making a diverting caecostomy. The post-operative course was uneventful but diarrhoea recurred as soon as feeding was resumed. Azidothymidine was introduced to no avail, and colonoscopy was repeated on July 21. The colon was still very inflamed. Biopsies showed characteristic nuclear CMV inclusions in endothelial cells, and a 3-week course of ganciclovir was administered, again to no avail. The patient's course went steadily downhill and a left lower quadrant colocutaneous fistula was found in September. A terminal ileostomy was performed. The patient died in October 1989. There was no autopsy.

Discussion

This patient had acquired immunodeficiency syndrome (AIDS) and her index AIDS disease according to the Centers for Disease Control (CDC) definition [1] was CMV colitis. Despite the lack of histological evidence, she probably already had CMV colitis in early May, and colon perforation in June. Mucosal biopsies have been shown to be positive in 92% of cases of well-documented CMV gastrointestinal disease, and rectal biopsies are positive in 80% of these cases [2]. So the negative initial biopsies do not rule out the possibility that our patient had CMV colitis in May. Standard histopathology is the best diagnostic test for gastrointestinal [2] mucosal CMV disease, and immunohistochemistry does not add significantly to its yield [2]. Rectal culture has a yield of only 30%, and urine culture is positive in 39%, but non-specific. Serum immunoglobulin G (IgG) and IgM levels are of no value [2].

CMV is a frequent pathogen in AIDS patients, causing active infection in 49%–90% of them [3–5]. In one series [3] it was the second most frequent pathogen, after *Pneumocystis carinii*. In this autopsy series of 164 patients, 81 had active CMV disease, with multiorgan involvement in 62%. The most frequently involved organs were the adrenals (75%; two deaths due to adrenal insufficiency), lungs (58%), gastrointestinal tract (30%), CNS (20%), eyes (10%), spleen (9%) and urinary tract (7%). CMV infection was responsible for death in 17 of these patients.

Gastrointestinal mucosal CMV disease can occur anywhere from the oesophagus to the rectum, causing a spectrum of disease ranging from nearly normal mucosa to severe inflammation with deep ulceration [2, 6]. Microscopically the characteristic CMV inclusions are typically seen in the nuclei of the endothelial cells. They can also occasionally be seen in epithelial cells towards the crypt base, and in macrophages and fibroblasts in the granulation tissue at the base of ulcers [2]. The rectum is the most commonly affected bowel segment [2, 6]. When biopsies are negative CMV colitis can be confused with ulcerative or granulomatous colitis [7] as in our patient. However if CMV colitis is suspected biopsies should be repeated [2].

Bowel perforation in gastrointestinal CMV disease has been reported in many cases [6–12], occurring in both the small and large bowel. Vasculitis due to preferential involvement of endothelial cells by CMV is thought to be responsible for ischaemia and perforation. In three reviews of AIDS patients who underwent surgery [7–10], bowel perforation due to CMV disease was noted in 7 out of 46 patients. It is thus a frequent cause of emergency surgery in these patients. The mean post-operative survival of the six patients who died was 2.7 months. In one series of AIDS patients who underwent emergency procedures (13 operations on 11 patients) CMV ileocolitis was responsible for 64% of the procedures and caused 70% of all deaths [7].

Treatment of gastrointestinal CMV disease is at best semi-satisfactory. Approximately three out of four patients treated with ganciclovir will respond to treatment with definite improvement in both their symptoms relative to CMV infection and their general well-being [5, 13, 14]. However, even with maintenance therapy following a 2-week induction course of ganciclovir, a large number of patients will relapse (with a median time to relapse of 8–9 weeks) and it has not been shown conclusively that ganciclovir therapy improves survival [14]. Furthermore some 10%–20% of patients show progressive disease despite induction therapy [13, 14]. The median survival of patients with CMV gastrointestinal disease treated with ganciclovir in one study was 4.5 months [14]. Ganciclovir treatment is often limited by toxicity: neutropenia or thrombopenia made it necessary to adjust dosage in one out of three patients in one series [14] and CNS toxicity (confusion or convulsions) was responsible for modifications of treatment in 11% of patients in another [4]. It would seem that CMV disease occurs in severely ill patients and that controlling its symptoms does not prevent the patient expiring from another opportunistic infection or neoplasm.

CMV and HIV may be synergistic co-pathogens. Skolnik et al. [15] have shown that cells experimentally infected with either virus are more susceptible to infection with the other. Furthermore HIV itself has been demonstrated in the epithelium, the lamina propria and the enterochromaffin cells of the bowel wall [16–19] and thus might be responsible for both the motility and malabsorption disorders in many AIDS patients. This phenomenon could be particularly important in the gastrointestinal tract which can be the portal of entry of both viruses in many AIDS patients.

AIDS patients may require surgery for conditions with no relation to HIV infection such as appendicitis. The post-operative morbidity and mortality in AIDS patients can be high, and this must be taken into account before proceeding to surgery. However, despite the high risk, many of these patients derive a true benefit from surgery, thus making the risk acceptable [8–11]. However, they more often undergo procedures for diseases which are related to their immune deficiency [8]. Elective procedures are commonly diagnostic, such as biopsies of lymph nodes, the lungs or retroperitoneal masses. Splenectomy can be required to treat refractory thrombocytopenia [9, 11].

Emergency procedures are required in some 3%–17% of AIDS patients for gastrointestinal haemorrhage, perforation or obstruction, all of which can be due to infectious diseases (notably CMV and MIC disease) or tumours (Kaposi's sarcoma or lymphomas). As previously discussed CMV disease can cause haemorrhage from ulceration anywhere in the gastrointestinal tract, and perforation of either small or large bowel. MIC disease can cause a Crohn's-like disease with intestinal obstruction [18]. Kaposi's sarcomas can either bleed or perforate [12].

High-grade extranodal B-cell lymphomas are frequently seen in AIDS patients [20], and can be the index AIDS disease [1]. In one report of 84 AIDS patients with lymphoma seven were in the gastrointestinal tract. The rectum was the most frequently involved area where these lesions can present as an abcess [20]. In other cases haemorrhage [9], obstruction or perforation can be the presenting symptom [8].

AIDS patients can also present with hepatobiliary disease due to CMV and/or *Cryptosporidium*. These agents can cause both a calculous cholecystitis and a peculiar from of sclerosing cholangitis [21, 22]. Papillary stenosis amenable to endoscopic sphincterotomy has also been described [23]. When this inflammatory process is localised mainly in the distal bile duct long-term relief of symptoms can be attained. When it is more diffuse the prognosis is poor. In one study [22], 12 out of 36 patients with CMV infection of the gastrointestinal tract or retinitis had cholestatic liver enzyme abnormalities which developed within 3 months of the diagnosis of CMV disease. Radiologic imaging showed dilatation in three out of nine patients who were studied. Ganciclovir therapy did not influence liver test results.

Anorectal disease is common in homosexual patients. When they develop AIDS and require surgery the outcome of surgery can be devastating. Wexner et al. [24] reported on 51 patients who underwent 73 procedures. Twenty-two patients were dead within 6 months with unhealed wounds; only six had satisfactory wound healing within 30 days and 17 required more than 6 months to heal. Other authors [25] have had less unsatisfactory results, but it would seem to be wise to avoid all anorectal surgery which is not absolutely necessary in these patients.

References

1. Centers for Disease Control (1987) Revision of the CDC surveillance case definition for Acquired Immunodeficiency Syndrome. MMWR 36 (suppl 1S): 3S–15S
2. Culpepper-Morgan JA, Kotler DP, Scholes JV, Tierney AR (1987) Evaluation of diagnostic criteria for mucosal cytomegalic inclusion disease in the Acquired Immune Deficiency Syndrome. Am J Gastroenterol 82: 1264–1270
3. Klatt EC, Shibata D (1988) Cytomegalovirus infection in the Acquired Immunodeficiency Syndrome. Clinical and autopsy findings. Arch Pathol Lab Med 112: 540–544
4. Drew WL (1988) Cytomegalovirus infection in patients with AIDS. J Infect Dis 158: 449–456
5. Jacobson MA, Mills J (1988) Serious cytomegalovirus disease in the Acquired Immunodeficiency Syndrome (AIDS). Clinical findings, diagnosis, and treatment. Ann Intern Med 108: 585–594
6. Rene E, Marche C, Chevalier T, Rouzioux C, Regnier B, Saimot AG, Negessey Y, Matheron S, Leport C, Wolff B, Moriniere B, Katlama C, Godeberge B, Vittecoq B, Bricaire F, Brun-Vesinet C, Pangon B, Dewol AM, Coulaud JP, Modai J, Frottier J, Vilde JL, Vachon F, Mignon M, Bonfils S (1988) Cytomegalovirus colitis in patients with Acquired Immunodeficiency Syndrome. Dig Dis Sci 33: 741–750
7. Wexner SD, Smithy WB, Trillo C, Smith Hopkins B, Dailey TH (1988) Emergency colectomy for cytomegalovirus ileocolitis in patients with the Acquired Immune Deficiency Syndrome. Dis Colon Rectum 31: 755–761
8. Macho JR (1988) Gastrointestinal surgery in the AIDS patient. Gastroenterol Clin North Am 17: 563–571
9. Ferguson CM (1988) Surgical complications of human immunodeficiency virus infection. Am Surg 54: 4–9
10. Robinson G, Wilson SE, Williams RA (1987) Surgery in patients with Acquired Immunodeficiency Syndrome. Arch Surg 122: 170–175
11. DeRiso AJ, Kemeny MM, Torres RA, Oliver JM (1989) Multiple jejunal perforations secondary to cytomegalovirus in a patient with Acquired Immune Deficiency Syndrome. Case report and review. Dig Dis Sci 34: 623–629
12. LaRaja RD, Rothenberg RE, Odom JW, Mueller SC (1989) The incidence of intra-abdominal surgery in Acquired Immunodeficiency Syndrome: a statistical review of 904 patients. Surgery 105: 175–179
13. Dieterich DT, Chachoua A, Lafleur F, Worrell C (1988) Ganciclovir treatment of gastrointestinal infections caused by cytomegalovirus in patients with AIDS. Rev Infect Dis 10: S532–537
14. Jacobson MA, O'Donnell JJ, Porteous D, Brodie HR, Feigal D, Mills J (1988) Retinal and gastrointestinal disease due to cytomegalovirus in patients with the Acquired Immune Deficiency Syndrome: prevalence, natural history, and response to ganciclovir therapy. QJ Med 254: 473–486
15. Skolnik PR, Kosloff BR, Hirsch MS (1988) Bidirectional interactions between human immunodeficiency virus type I and cytomegalovirus. J Infect Dis 157: 508–514
16. Nelson JA, Reynolds-Kohler C, Margaretten W, Wiley CA, Reese CE, Levy JA (1988) Human immunodeficiency virus detected in bowel epithelium from patients with gastrointestinal symptoms. Lancet I: 259–262
17. Ullrich R, Zeitz M, Heise W, L'age M, Höffken G, Riecken EO (1989) Small intestinal structure and function in patients infected with human immunodeficiency virus (HIV): evidence for HIV-induced enteropathy. Ann Intern Med 111: 15–21
18. Fox CH, Kotler D, Tierney A, Wilson CS, Fauci AS (1989) Detection of HIV-1 RNA in the lamina propria of patients with AIDS and gastrointestinal disease. J Infect Dis 159: 467–471
19. Levy JA, Margaretten W, Nelson J (1989) Detection of HIV in enterochromaffin cells in the rectal mucosa of an AIDS patient. Am J Gastroenterol 84: 787–789

20. Kaplan LD, Abrams DI, Feigal E, McGrath M, Kahn J, Neville P, Ziegler J, Volberding PA (1989) AIDS-associated non-Hodgkin's lymphoma in San Francisco. JAMA 261: 719–724
21. Margulis SJ, Honig CL, Soave R, Govoni AF, Mouradian JA, Jacobson IM (1986) Biliary tract obstruction in the Acquired Immunodeficiency Syndrome. Ann Intern Med 105: 207–210
22. Jacobson MA, Cello JP, Sande MA (1988) Cholestasis and disseminated cytomegalovirus disease in patients with the Acquired Immunodeficiency Syndrome. Am J Med 84: 218–224
23. Schneidermann DJ, Cello JP, Laing FC (1987) Papillary stenosis and sclerosing cholangitis in the Acquired Immunodeficiency Syndrome. Ann Intern Med 106: 546–549
24. Wexner SD, Smithy WB, Milsom JW, Dailey TH (1986) The surgical management of anorectal diseases in AIDS and pre-AIDS patients. Dis Colon Rectum 29: 719–723
25. Barone JE, Wolkomir AF, Muakkassa FF, Fares LG (1988) Abdominal pain and anorectal disease in AIDS. Gastroenterol Clin North Am 17: 631–638

Condylomata Acuminata in HIV-Positive Patients: Recent Results of a Prospective Ongoing Study

P. Buchmann, D. Christen, R. Grob, H.P. Simmen and R. Rüdlinger

Introduction

Condylomata acuminata (anogenital warts) are caused by human papilloma viruses (HPV) of different types [9]. In many patients there is a history of sexual transmission although others are unable to remember a contact with a possible risk. Some patients attend our proctological clinic, run by surgeons, of their own accord; others, mainly with extensive disease, are referred for therapy.

In 1986 we started to register all our patients with condylomata acuminata and to test them for human immunodeficiency virus (HIV) infection because we had observed that in HIV-positive patients condylomata were much more extensive.

Not long ago we presented the results relating to the first 23 patients [4]. We stressed that the two-step operation recommended by some authors for very extensive lesions gives poor results in HIV-positive patients. A week or two after surgery, the affected area looked the same as it did before treatment or even worse. Therefore we suggest radical treatment for all patients in the first instance. We concluded further that 70% of our patients with condylomata acuminata were HIV-positive, and that the recurrence rate was equal in patients with or without HIV infection, although in HIV-positive patients recurrence occurred earlier and was more extensive. Postoperative complications were seen only in stage IV infection. In the meantime the number of patients has increased threefold justifying a new analysis of the series.

Patients and Methods

Between July 1986 and December 1989 all patients presenting with condylomata acuminata at the proctological clinic of the University Hospital, Zurich, were asked about homosexuality, intravenous drug abuse and HIV-related diseases. If no HIV test had been done previously, a serological test (enzyme-linked immunosorbent assay, ELISA, and western

Table 1. Sex distribution and age of patients

	Whole patient group	HIV-positive	HIV-negative
Total number of patients (n)	67	38[a]	29
Male (n)	57	34	23
Female (n)	10	4	6
Age (years)			
Mean (range)	28(21–50)	31(18–61)	

[a] Totalled 57% of all patients

Table 2. Risk factors of HIV-positive (n = 38) and HIV-negative (n = 29) patients

Risk	All patients	HIV+	HIV−
None	21	2*	19*
Homosexual	30	21	9
IV drug abuser	12	12	0
Both homosexual and i.v. drug abuser	4	3	1

* $p < 0.001$

blot) was performed. Classification of HIV-related disease was done according to the Centers for Disease Control (CDC) system [5]. Local spread of condylomata was scored according to a grading system applied separately to the "outside" ranging from the perianal region to the dentate line and to the "inside" encompassing the dentate line and the rectal mucosa above it. We scored one asterisk (*) for a single condylomata of up to several millimetres in size, two asterisks (**) for multiple but not confluent lesions, three asterisks (***) for widespread, partially confluent lesions and four asterisks (****) for circular and extended cushions of condylomata. In some patients HPV was identified by Southern hybridisation analysis [9].

For the majority of patients treatment included an operation. After injection of a vasoconstrictive drug (Por 8, Sandoz, Switzerland, 1 unit Por 8 to 20 units physiologic saline) under the lesion, large condylomata from "outside" were removed using scissors, and smaller lesions were electrocoagulated. In the case of extended lesions on the mucous membrane a large biopsy was taken and the remaining condylomata were treated by extensive electrocoagulation. (At the beginning of the study a few HIV positive patients with very large lesions were treated in two stages, previously a routine procedure. However, during the first two postoperative weeks huge recurrences were observed, leading to a change in therapeutic regime). Special care to leave large vital skin bridges between excisional wounds was taken only in the outer anal canal between the anocutaneous line and the dentate line. Post operative assessments were made weekly initially and monthly after 4 weeks. A patient was judged to be cured after

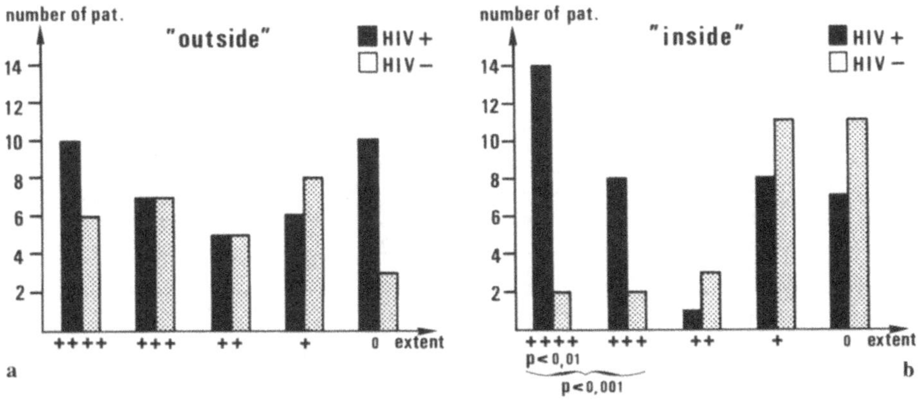

Fig. 1. Local spread of condylomata for **a** outside lesions and **b** inside lesions. +, single condylomata of up to several millimeters; ++, multiple but not confluent lesions; +++, widespread, partially confluent lesions; ++++, circular, extended cushians of condylomata

a 3-month interval without recurrence. Large recurrences were removed surgically; smaller ones were treated with podophyllin (4%).

Over a 2½-year period 67 patients, 10 female and 57 male, were included in our study. Their mean age was 29 years (Table 1). Thirty-eight (57%) were infected with HIV, i.e. seropositive. As shown in Table 2, 30 were homosexual, 12 were intravenous drug addicts and four were both of these. Only 21 had no such risk, two in the seropositive and 19 in the seronegative group ($p < 0.001$). Among the HIV-positive patients 17 were classified grade II, 11 grade III and 10 grade IV. The pre-treatment scoring for local spread of condylomata is shown in Fig. 1 for outside and inside lesions. There was no difference between seropositive and seronegative patients with regard to the extent of condylomata in the outside region, whereas with regard to the inside region a significantly higher number of HIV-positive patients demonstrated large lesions ($p < 0.01$). Subdivision of the scoring into the three CDC classification stages is shown in Table 3. The stage of HIV infection does not indicate the extent of the disease.

Statistical significance was calculated by Chi-square test or by Wilcoxon's rank-som test.

Results

Reviewing average natural history of condylomata acuminata, the time from onset to the first visit to the doctor was twice as long in seropositive patients (mean 12 months, range 1 month to over a year) than it was in seronegative patients (mean 6 months, range 3–12 months). Of the 67 patients, 62 were

Table 3. Subdivision of scoring of extent of condylomata acuminata in HIV positive patients into CDC classification stages

Score	Outside			Inside		
	II	III	IV	II	III	IV
****	6	2	2	6	4	4
***	4	2	1	4	2	2
**	3	–	2	–	–	1
*	3	2	1	4	2	2
Nil	1	5	4	3	3	1
Total	17	11	10	17	11	10

Table 4. Condyloma recurrence and HIV infection

Frequency of recurrence	HIV-positive (n = 34)	HIV-negative (n = 28)
1	13	11
2	4	4
3	–	5

Table 5. Localisation of recurrences

Frequency of recurrence	HIV-positive (n = 34)		HIV-negative (n = 28)	
	Outside	Inside	Outside	Inside
1	9	9	8	7
2	3	1	4	2
3	–	–	4	1

surgically treated, 34 seropositive and 28 seronegative. One patient with HIV stage IV and one seronegative patient with minor lesions were treated nonoperatively. The remaining two positive patients (stage II and III) did not attend the proposed operation. Another patient (stage IV) did not attend after therapy. So three patients were lost for follow-up. Thirty-four HIV-seropositive and 28 seronegative patients remained for postoperative evaluation.

At least one recurrence was seen in 13 out of 34 HIV-positive patients and 11 out of 28 HIV negative patients (Table 4). The localisation of recurrences is shown in Table 5. Although up to three recurrences were observed in seronegative patients, the extent of these repeated recurrences

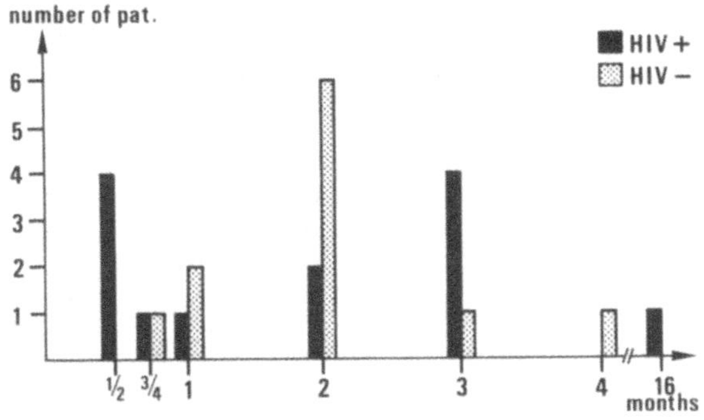

Fig. 2. Interval between initial operation and first recurrence

Table 6. Number of recurrences and operations needed to clear all condylomata acuminata

Number of operations	HIV-positive (n = 34)		HIV-negative (n = 28)	
	Recurrence (n)	Operation needed (n)	Recurrence (n)	Operation needed (n)
1	–	23[a]	–	17[b]
2	13	7	11	8
3	4	4	4	2
4	0	0	5	1

[a] 60%
[b] 58%

Table 7. Interval between second operation and second recurrence

Weeks	HIV-positive (n = 13)	HIV-negative (n = 11)
2	1	1
4	–	2
8	1	–
12	1	1
36	1	–

was small in the majority as indicated by the number of operations needed for cure (Table 6).

The interval between the initial operation and the first recurrence is shown is Fig. 2. In seropositive patients recurrences were observed earlier than in the seronegative group. However, this did not reach a level of significance, and second recurrences did not demonstrate this difference either (Table 7).

Table 8. Postoperative complications

	Total number of patients	Complication	No. of patients affected
HIV-negative	28	None	None
HIV-positive			
Stage II	16	None	None
III	10	Abscess	1
IV	8	Delayed healing	1
		Abscess	1
		Phlegmon	1

No postoperative complications were seen in seronegative and seropositive stage II patients (Table 8). Two out of ten patients with stage III infection (20%) developed a complication. In one of these an abscess formation caused by a fistula 5 mm distally from the dentate line was found 3 months after the first operation. Deroofing and fistulotomy was followed by a prolonged inflammatory infiltration of the skin surrounding the wound which required antibiotic treatment. With this therapy the wound healed within 4 weeks. The second patient demonstrated delayed wound healing.

Two out of eight patients with HIV infection stage IV developed infection. One of them had an intersphincteric abscess which spread to the perianal region within 2 weeks after removal of the condylomata; he was operated on and antibiotics were given concomitantly. The postoperative course was uneventful. The other patient developed a perianal phlegmon 2 months postoperatively which was cured with antibiotics. There was no rebleeding or stenosis requiring intervention. Histological examination of the biopsies was always negative for carcinoma. HPV types found in the condylomata are given in Table 9.

Discussion

To our knowledge no other group has to date published a report which deals with condylomata acuminata in patients with acquired immunodeficiency syndrome (AIDS). Although in recent years the literature on AIDS has been increasing day by day, proctological problems are rarely discussed, except for the high rate of malignant tumours among homosexual males [8, 11] and proctitis related to viral infection or gay bowel syndrome [3, 9].

In the summer of 1986 we started to follow all HIV-positive patients with proctological disorders and published our first report in 1988 [6]. Of the 27 patients included, 18 were suffering from condylomata acuminata. In the summer of 1986 we also began HIV-serological testing for all patients who presented with condylomata acuminata at the proctological clinic of the

Table 9. Results of HPV Southern hybridisation analysis in 28 patients

HPV type	HIV-positive (n = 16) Stage			HIV-negative (n = 12)
	II	III	IV	
6	5	2	1	7
11	1	4	3	2
6 or 11[a]				3

[a] Type not further determined

University Hospital Zurich. In a recent paper we stated that 70% of patients were seropositive and that there was only one woman in 16 patients [4]. In the most recent data, with 67 patients, this percentage is reduced to 57% and the male to female ratio is 34:4 (Table 1). This ratio for males is, nevertheless, very high when compared with the European AIDS patients' male to female ratio of 1.4:1 [1]. One reason may be that in our series intravenous drug addicts are more frequent (42%) than in the average European AIDS population (30%) as are homosexuals (approximately 55% compared with 49% in Europe) [1]. A highly significant difference in patients with risk factors can be demonstrated between seropositive and seronegative patients ($p < 0.001$, Table 2). Lesions were scored to allow comparison of the two groups. There was no difference found in the spread of condylomata outside the anus and up to the dentate line, although on the mucous membrane a significantly increased number of seropositive patients demonstrated circular cushions as far as 3 cm into the rectal ampulla (Fig. 1). This was irrespective of the severity of symptoms of HIV infection (Table 3). There are two possible explanations for this observation. Firstly, resistance to HPV in seropositive patients may be less in the rectal mucosa than distally at the dentate line. This, however, does not seem to be the case because the data shown in Table 3 do not indicate an increased growth of condylomata in patients with stage III and stage IV HIV infection. Furthermore septic complications do not originate from this location (Table 8). A second explanation might relate to contamination by anal intercourse. This might be more likely since there are about 13% homosexuals in the seronegative group and about 55% in the seropositive group of patients (Table 2). No real difference in HPV type was found although there seems to be a predominance of HPV 6 in HIV negative patients (Table 9). No malignancy-associated HPV-type was detected and the pattern (HPV 6 and 11) is the same as that in the general population [9]. This observation does not contradict the fact that infections with high-risk HPV types seem to be particularly prevalent among HIV-positive homosexuals [2], since their lesions were not of condylomata acuminata type. Our histological findings which show no signs of malignant or premalignant change even in very extensive lesions support this assumption.

Somewhat disappointing in this series is the recurrence rate which is about the same in both groups (Table 4). This is difficult to understand in the seronegative patients. There was no difference in the distribution of lesions outside or inside the anal canal (Table 5). However, the time interval between the operation and first recurrence was slightly less in HIV-positive patients (Fig. 2), although in second recurrences no such difference could be demonstrated (Table 7). Our hypothesis to explain this observation is difficult to prove. In HIV-positive patients a viral infection immediately creates a visible condyloma. By contrast, in seronegative patients there might be a number of "dormant" viruses which cause new condylomata after treatment. This theory is supported by our impression that recurrent condylomata in HIV-negative patients are smaller in size and number. Recurrences do not always need surgical treatment for cure (Table 6). However, all four second recurrences in seropositive patients were surgically treated (Tables 4 and 6). In seronegative patients only two out of four patients who had two recurrences and one out of five who had three recurrences needed further operations. In the other two, and four patients respectively, the lesions were so small that treatment with podophyllin was sufficient.

No complications were seen in HIV-seronegative and stage II seropositive patients (Table 8). We already stressed 2 years ago that complications arise in half of all stage IV patients treated [6]. In the two later stages of HIV infection the complication rate is rather high. However, the percentage has decreased considerably. All infections originated from the lower anal canal and delayed wound healing was observed in the same location. Where deroofing of an abscess was necessary, healing sometimes required additional antibiotic therapy. We therefore emphasise the benefit of prophylactic antibiotics for patients with stage III and IV HIV infection during removal of condylomata acuminata, similar to the practice we employ in all other proctological interventions [6]. However, as mentioned in our report [6] we question the need for bowel preparation preceding an anal operation. Before referral to our clinic some of the seropositive patients were treated with alpha-2-recombinate interferon without success. This confirms the observation made by other authors that this drug is not especially effective in the treatment of HIV-infected patients [7].

Although about 40% of our patients needed more than one intervention, we still believe that our one-stage procedure is an adequate therapy for condylomata acuminata. Podophyllin helps in the case of very small lesions, especially in recurrences.

References

1. AIDS Surveillance in Europe (1989) Quarterly report N° 22, June 30th. European Center for the epidemiological monitoring of AIDS, St Maurice, France
2. Barrasso R, De Brux J, Croissant O, Orth G (1987) High prevalence of papilloma virus-associated penile intraepithelial neoplasia in sexual partners of women with cervical intraepithelial neoplasia. N Engl J Med 317: 916–923
3. Buchmann P, Täuber MG (1988) HIV-Infektion und proktologische Erkrankungen. In: Buchmann P (ed) Lehrbuch der Proktologie. Huber, Bern, pp 211–218
4. Buchmann P, Christen D, Rüdlinger R, Geroulanos S (1991) Anale Condylomata acuminata. Ein prospektiver Vergleich von HIV-positiven und -negativen Patienten. Chirurg 62: 32–35
5. Centers for Disease Control (1986) Classification system for human T-lymphotropic virus type III/lymphadenopathy-associated virus infections. MMWR 35: 334–339
6. Christen D, Buchmann P, Rüdlinger R (1988) Verlauf proktologischer Affektionen beim HIV-positiven Patienten. Schweiz Rundsch Med Prax 44: 1208–1211
7. Douglas JM, Rogers M, Judson FN (1986) The effect of asymptomatic infection with HTLV-III on the response of anogenital warts to intralesional treatment with recombinant alpha-2-interferon. J Infect Dis 154: 331–334
8. Peters RK, Mack TM (1983) Patterns of anal carcinoma by gender and marital status in Los Angeles County. Br J Cancer 48: 629–636
9. Rüdlinger R (1988) Warzen im äusseren Anogenitalbereich, unter spezieller Berücksichtigung von HIV-positiven Patienten. Schweiz Rundsch Med Prax 77: 1202–1207
10. Rüdlinger R, Grob R, Buchmann P, Christen D, Steiner R (1988) Anogenital warts of the condyloma acuminata type in HIV-positive patients. Dermatologica 176: 277–281
11. Rüdlinger R, Buchmann P (1989) HIV 16-positive bowenoid papulosis and squamous-cell carcinoma of the anus in an HIV-positive Man. Dis Colon Rectum 32: 1042–1045

Ten Years of Colorectal Surgery in Chur: Audit and Training

A. Fiennes, C. Ryf, N. Renz, M. Furrer, T. Rüedi and A. Leutenegger

Introduction

The Cantonal Hospital in Chur serves an area with 750 patients per doctor. The canton is the largest but least densely populated in Switzerland and, apart from some peripheral hospitals, its resident population of 175 000 is served by a surgical service of two trained surgeons and three chief assistants. We have sought evidence for an effect of this structure on the workload distribution, quality of care and training potential attached to surgery of the colon and rectum, with particular reference to colorectal carcinoma.

Methods

Case records were examined retrospectively for all operations performed on the colon in the past 10 years (1980–1989). Of a total of 557 operations, 553 records were suitable for further analysis. Among these were 321 operations for carcinoma of the colon or rectum. This subset of records was examined for demographic details, complications, hospital stay, death and ascertained cause, location of tumour, tumour stage, operation and operator. Details of operation category (emergency or elective), antibiotic and antiembolic treatment and of operative technique were also collected.

Results

Demography, Morbidity and Mortality

The average age of patients undergoing an aggregate of 321 operations for colorectal carcinoma was 66.8 years (standard deviation 12.3 years). Forty per cent were women, and a total of 149 operations were complicated

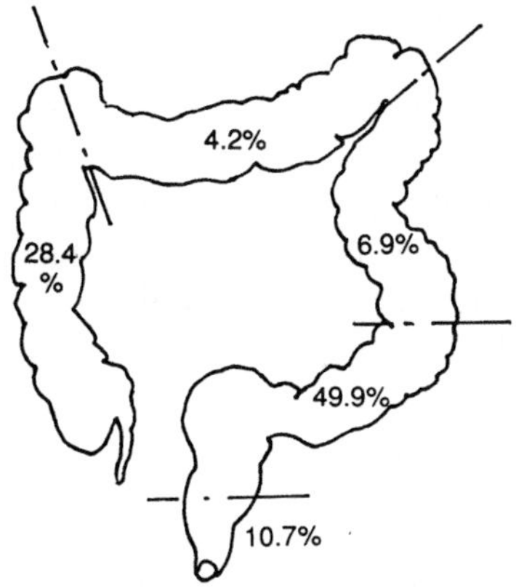

Fig. 1. Distribution of colorectal carcinomas around the bowel in 321 cases

peri- or post-operatively (46%). Mean hospital stay was 27 days (standard deviation 17 days) and 18 patients died in hospital in the wake of an operation, a crude operative mortality of 5.6%.

Distribution of Tumours

Approximately one third of tumours were proximal to the splenic flexure and two thirds were in the left colon, sigmoid colon or rectum and anal canal. Among the resections performed there were a total of 4.5% Dukes stage A, 16% stage B1, 30% B2 (total stage B 46%), 4.2% stage C1 and 26.8% C2 (total C 31%). The remainder of resections were in patients with metastases.

Operator, Class of Operation and Mortality

Just 22 of 321 operations (7%) were classed as emergencies. Fully trained surgeons operated electively on 195 patients with five deaths and on 15 emergencies with one death. For chief assistants the figures were 101 (eight deaths) and 7 (three deaths), respectively. One death occurred in a patient of unclassified operation category. There was no significant difference in the proportion of emergency operations undertaken by the two groups of surgeon, nor in their mortality rates for elective or emergency operating respectively. These categories as a whole were also associated with statistically indistinguishable mortality rates. No operation was undertaken by an unsupervised trainee of lower grade.

Cause of Death and Complications

Pulmonary embolus accounted for more deaths (5/17) than any other cause, followed by circulatory failure (4/17) and multiorgan failure (3/17). Complications were equally distributed between surgeons, irrespective of rank. Wound infection was the commonest problem, occurring after 9.7% of all operations. This frequency was only rivalled by deep vein thrombosis and pulmonary embolus, which ensued from 5.4% of operations.

Anastomotic Leak

Leaks occurred after a total of 11 operations and one was associated with postoperative death. None of the leaking anastomoses had been protected by defunctioning stoma and six of the eight leaks that resulted from anterior resection were from stapled anastomoses. This finding is of borderline significance, since overall just half the 82 anterior resections had stapled anastomoses ($0.05 < p < 0.1$).

Discussion

Our patient cohort is comparable to those reported by other authors in terms of age and sex distribution, but the crude operative mortality, from which early cancer-related deaths have not been separated, is unusually low [1, 2]. There were exceptionally few emergency operations and the distribution of tumour stage shows more tumours confined to the bowel than in larger UK series [3]. The latter data may reflect a relatively high standard of primary care in general practice, as befits a mountainous region with many isolated communities. There was no statistical evidence that operation by a surgeon in training conferred a higher mortality.

The reported complication rate may seem high, but only half the reports specify a given complication. This may reflect the application of high standards to case note review and highlights the difficulties of retrospective grading.

The overall complication rate was not related to individual operators or groups of operator. Thus there was no evidence that operation by a surgeon in training conferred an overall higher morbidity: no operation was undertaken by an unsupervised junior below chief assistant grade.

However the aggregate frequency of lethal and non-lethal thromboembolic complications was significantly greater among chief assistants. If this is interpreted as reflecting increased operating time due to inexperience, then increasing the proportion of surgery undertaken by trainees might reduce rather than increase morbidity and mortality, unless training is to cease altogether. In the Bath study [2] there was no significant difference in morbidity or mortality between chiefs and trainees, although there the latter undertook a greater proportion of surgery than those in Chur and were often of less senior rank.

We did not find any literature with which to compare our figure of 27 days for mean in-patient stay.

It is not certain that low stapled anastomoses were more likely to leak than those sutured by hand. However, the findings in this study may promote a greater willingness to defunction low anastomoses by caecostomy.

References

1. Lockhart-Mummery HE, Ritchie JK, Hawley PR (1976) The results of surgical treatment for carcinoma of the rectum at St. Mark's Hospital from 1948 to 1972. Br J Surg 63: 673–677
2. Chester J, Britton D (1989) Elective and emergency surgery for colorectal cancer in a district general hospital: impact of surgical training on patient survival. Ann R Coll Surg Engl 71: 370–374
3. Umpleby HC, Bristol JB, Rainey JB, Williamson RC (1984) Survival of 727 patients with single carcinomas of the large bowel. Dis Col Rect 27: 803–810

Abnormalities of the Neural Control of the Internal Anal Sphincter in Idiopathic Faecal Incontinence

C.T.M. Speakman, C.H.V. Hoyle, M.A. Kamm, M.M. Henry, R.J. Nicholls and G. Burnstock

Introduction

Over the past 10 years histological studies and neurophysiological techniques have increased our understanding of the pathophysiology of idiopathic faecal incontinence [1–7]. It is now believed that damage to the somatic innervation of the striated external anal sphincter and puborectalis muscles leads to progressive weakness. However, there is increasing evidence that in a proportion of patients with idiopathic faecal incontinence the internal anal sphincter (IAS) is also abnormal. Studies of patients with faecal incontinence have shown that the maximum resting anal pressure, which is mainly produced by internal sphincter activity [8–10], is abnormally low [4, 11] and that there is fibrosis and atrophy of the IAS in patients with neurogenic incontinence [12, 13]. One theory is that these changes may be due to damage to the innervation of the IAS [12] and we have tested this by analyzing the in vitro response of the internal anal sphincter to noradrenaline, an important sympathetic neurotransmitter in the IAS, and to electrical field stimulation (EFS), which is known to stimulate the intrinsic nerves in the IAS [14].

Subjects

Twelve patients undergoing postanal repair were studied. They all suffered with incontinence to solid stool. There were 11 women and 1 man. Of the 11 women, eight had previously had forceps delivery and five described having prolonged deliveries. The mean age of the incontinent group was 54 years (range 32–79 years).

Ten patients undergoing abdomino-perineal excision for low rectal carcinoma were studied as controls. There were four female patients and six males, mean age 59 years (range 44–82 years). None of the controls had a history of faecal incontinence.

Methods

All incontinent subjects underwent preoperative anorectal physiology. Maximum resting anal pressure and maximum voluntary contraction pressures were measured using a closed water-filled system with a 4 mm diameter microballoon [2]. Assessment of the state of innervation of the striated pelvic floor muscles was performed using measurement of pudendal nerve terminal motor latencies and single fibre electromyography of the external anal sphincter. These methods have been described previously [1, 3].

A 10 mm long by 3 mm wide circumferential strip of the IAS was taken during the intersphincteric dissection of postanal repair and placed into Krebs' solution. The control tissue was taken from the resected abdomino-perineal specimen, removing the most distal strip of the IAS.

From the tissue removed, two to four strips were dissected under a microscope and suspended in 3- or 5-ml organ baths containing modified Krebs' solution at 37°C and perfused with 95% O_2 and 5% CO_2. Contraction and relaxation responses were recorded via transducers on a Grass polygraph. Noradrenaline was added to the organ baths in increasing concentrations (10^{-8}–10^{-4} *M*) until the maximum contraction had been obtained. Phentolamine (10^{-6} *M*), an alpha blocker, was then added to the Krebs' solution and, noradrenaline was again added in increasing concentrations. From the responses obtained the concentrations required to produce maximum response and 50% of maximum, the EC_{50}, were calculated.

Two platinum ring electrodes immersed in the organ bath were used to produce electrical field stimulation (EFS). Responses to a range of stimuli (1–32 Hz) were recorded using stimulation of 150 V and pulse duration of 0.5 ms.

Results

Anorectal Physiology

The mean resting anal pressure was 30 cm H_2O (normal range 40–100 cm H_2O), the mean maximum voluntary contraction pressure was 30 cm H_2O (normal range 40–160 cm H_2O). Pudendal nerve latencies were prolonged in all patients, and single fibre density was raised. These results indicate that the patients studied had neurogenic faecal incontinence with poorly functioning IAS and external anal sphincters.

In Vitro Responses

Noradrenaline. The muscle strips from both the controls and the incontinent patients contracted to noradrenaline. When phentolamine was added to the Krebs' solution, noradrenaline caused relaxations. This relaxation could be blocked by the addition of propranolol, a beta-blocker. This shows that the contraction is an alpha-adrenoreceptor-mediated response, and the relaxation, a beta response. The concentration of noradrenaline required to produce a given response (proportion of maximum contraction) was higher in the incontinent group of patients than in the controls at each concentration tested, but there was no significant difference between the concentration-response curves when phentolamine, an alpha-blocker, was added to the perfusing solution.

Electrical Field Stimulation. The muscle strips responded to EFS by relaxations. After the addition of phentolamine, the relaxations were significantly larger in the control group, but not in the incontinent group.

Discussion

In this study we have demonstrated a decreased sensitivity to the noradrenaline in idiopathic faecal incontinence which is due to an abnormality of the alpha-adrenoreceptors. We have also shown that there is an alpha-adrenergic effect on the intrinsic innervation which is abnormal in incontinence. The IAS receives a dense extrinsic sympathetic innervation [15] which is most likely to exert a contractile response [16–18]. Our findings of decreased sensitivity to an important sympathetic neurotransmitter therefore suggest a possible sympathetic denervation in idiopathic faecal incontinence. This would be in keeping with the in vivo findings of changes in the frequency and duration of the spontaneous IAS relaxations [19, 20] and the reduced frequency of EMG recorded slow-wave activity in faecal incontinence. It is possible that a clearer understanding of the pharmacological abnormalities of the IAS in incontinence may lead to development of new therapies in the management of idiopathic faecal incontinence.

References

1. Parks AG, Swash M, Urich H (1977) Sphincter denervation in anorectal incontinence and rectal prolapse. Gut 18: 656–665
2. Beersiek F, Parks AG, Swash M (1979) Pathogenesis of ano-rectal incontinence. A histometric study of the anal sphincter musculature. J Neurol Sci 42: 111–127
3. Neill ME, Swash M (1980) Increased motor unit fibre density in the external anal sphincter muscle in ano-rectal incontinence: a single fibre EMG study. J Neurol Neurosurg Psychiatry 43: 343–347
4. Neill ME, Parks AG, Swash M (1981) Physiological studies of the anal sphincter musculature in faecal incontinence and rectal prolapse. Br J Surg 68: 531–536
5. Kiff ES, Swash M (1984) Slowed conduction in the pudendal nerves in idiopathic (neurogenic) faecal incontinence. Br J Surg 71: 614–616
6. Bartolo DC, Jarratt JA, Read MG, Donnelly TC, Read NW (1983) The role of partial denervation of the puborectalis muscle in idiopathic faecal incontinence. Br J Surg 70: 664–667
7. Womack NR, Morrison JF, Williams NS (1986) The role of pelvic floor denervation in the aetiology of idiopathic faecal incontinence. Br J Surg 73: 404–407
8. Duthie HL, Watts JM (1965) Contribution of the external anal sphincter to the pressure zone in the anal canal. Gut 6: 64–68
9. Frenckner B, von Euler C (1975) Influence of pudendal block on the function of the anal sphincters. Gut 16: 482–489
10. Lestar B, Penninckx F, Kerremans R. (1989) The composition of anal basal pressure. An in vivo and in vitro study in man. Int J Colorect Dis 4: 118–122
11. Sun WM, Read NW, Donnelly TC (1989) Impaired internal anal sphincter in a subgroup of patients with idiopathic fecal incontinence. Gastroenterology 97: 130–135
12. Lubowski DZ, Nicholls RJ, Burleigh DE, Swash M (1988) Internal anal sphincter in neurogenic fecal incontinence. Gastroenterology 95: 997–1002
13. Swash M, Gray A, Lubowski DZ, Nicholls RJ (1988) Ultrastructural changes in internal anal sphincter in neurogenic faecal incontinence. Gut 29: 1692–1698
14. Burleigh DE, D'Mello A, Parks AG (1979) Responses of isolated human internal anal sphincter to drugs and electrical field stimulation. Gastroenterology 77: 484–490
15. Baumgarten HG, Holstein AF, Stelzner F (1971) Differences in the innervation of the large intestine and internal anal sphincter in mammals and humans. Verh Anat Ges 66: 43–47
16. Rankin FW, Learmonth JR (1930) Section of sympathetic nerves of distal part of colon and rectum in treatment of Hirschsprung's disease and certain types of constipation. Ann Surg 92: 710–720
17. Carlstedt A, Nordgren S, Fasth S, Appelgren L, Hulten L (1988) Sympathetic nervous influence on the internal anal sphincter and rectum in man. Int J Colorect Dis 3: 90–95
18. Frenckner B, Ihre T (1976) Influence of autonomic nerves on the internal anal sphincter in man. Gut 17: 306–312
19. Kumar D, Waldron DL, Williams NS (1989) Home assessment of anorectal motility and external sphincter EMG in idiopathic faecal incontinence. Br J Surg 76: 635
20. Sun WM, Read NW, Miner PB, Kerrigan DD, Donnelly TC (1990) The role of transient internal sphincter relaxation in faecal incontinence? Int J Colorect Dis 5: 31–36

Part VI: Round Tables

How Is Rectal Cancer Best Managed?

R.J. Heald, P.F. Schofield, J. Pettavel, and R. Mirimanoff

Controversies in Current Surgical Management

R.J. Heald

Our President, Mr Geoffrey Oates, has recently reviewed the management of rectal cancer in a most articulate manner in his Presidential Address – "Rectal Carcinoma: do we need to be so gloomy?" I will therefore try to avoid repeating the crucial points which he then made, except to restate the fundamental point that rectal carcinoma requires specialised and experienced surgeons. The surgical agenda at each operation will be the total excision of the rectum with its integral visceral mesentery, the mesorectum, and our President specifically emphasised the need to guard against implantation by cross clamping and washout. There remain, however, three clear areas of controversy in the actual surgical management which I will endeavour to address today.

How Low Dare We Go?

It is interesting that the current graphs for abdominoperineal excision and anterior resection at St Mark's Hospital appear to be converging rather than diverging. It thus appears that almost one half of all rectal adenocarcinoma patients at St Mark's Hospital are now being offered abdominoperineal excision. The graph of these trends over the years at St Mark's Hospital is well known to us all, and the present figure shows only a slight predominance of anterior resection.

A small paper in the *British Journal of Surgery* entitled "The Close Shave in Anterior Resection" presents the results of our attempts at Basingstoke to perform the maximum possible number of anterior resections in a series of 230 cases analysed at the beginning of last year. The incidence of abdominoperineal excision has been reduced to 9%. We identified 42% in whom the preservation of the anal sphincter dictated the reduction of the distal muscle tube margin (not including the staple doughnut) to 1 cm or less. If we were to add this "close shave" group to our abdominoperineal excision group, our own percentage for abdominoperitoneal excisions would come up to around 40%, so it is perhaps interesting to analyse what price has been exacted from the patients for this decision to conserve their anal sphincters. It is interesting and surprising to find that not one single local recurrence has yet been detected in the 42 "close shave" cases. All four of the local recurrences that we had detected at the time of preparing these figures had occurred in the conventional margin group, and I can add on this occasion that the two further local recurrences that we have since detected were also in the conventional margin group. At the 95% confidence limits this represents a possible range of 0–5.9% in the "close shave" group and 0.8%–7.4% in the conventional margin group. Both of these groups were of course in patients classified as potentially curable. The possibility that a greater margin might confer any benefit is thus infinitesimally small. Similarly favourable results were, surprisingly, found in terms of distant metastases, since the "close shave" group had a 10% metastasis rate compared with a 14.6% metastases rate in the conventional group. The explanation for these differences must have been mostly a question of chance, although there were 35% of Dukes A cases in the "close shave" group in comparison with 17.3% in the conventional group. In my opinion this reflected our tendency to avoid "close shave" cases with larger infiltrating tumours, and there is clearly a greater willingness to go closer to the lower edge of a more favourable lesion.

The question of anastomotic leakage in these lower anastomoses was recently addressed by me at the Presidential Meeting in Birmingham, and I will not repeat what I then said. Anastomotic leakage does, however, remain a refractory problem both in my own hands and I understand also in the hands of all the surgeons at St Mark's Hospital. For this reason it has been my continued policy to protect the ultralow anastomosis with a temporary loop transverse colostomy.

The Anterior Plane in Cancer

For a number of years it has been my policy to identify the plane between the seminal vesicles and Denonvillier's fascia anterior to the middle third of the rectum and to dissect down to the point where Denonvillier's fascia becomes fused to the back of the prostate. In most cases this point of fusion, which must be divided transversely, will take one clear of the common middle-third rectal carcinoma. In this way, Denonvillier's fascia may be removed with the specimen and an extra safety margin of mesorectal tissue thus excised. At a recent panel discussion in the United States, Victor Fazio expressed the view that this was a dangerous practice which would result in autonomic nerve damage. I do not believe that this necessarily follows, provided that the presacral nerves have been identified and followed forwards as far as the lateral extremities of Denonvillier's fascia, and the fascia is excised like a "bib" on the front of the rectum with converging sides so that its lower extremity is a good deal narrower than its upper one. The nerves themselves are carefully left within the patient and great pains are taken to avoid "taking the tops off" these vital structures. I believe that the question of the anterior plane in middle-third carcinoma would be a useful area for debate at this meeting.

The Significance of Lateral Margin Involvement

A recent paper in *The Lancet* from Guildford – in some ways a published version of papers presented at the tripartite meeting of our own section last year – raised two important points regarding the histopathology of the mesorectum. John Nicholls, at our meeting to celebrate the life of Sir Hugh Lockhart-Mummery, drew our attention to the limitations of the histopathological staging as the "big step" towards an adverse prognosis that the Dukes staging system implies. The Guildford group pointed out that a substantial direct mesorectal spread of more than 4 mm represented a larger and more significant step than the involvement of a lymph node. The accompanying editorial also pointed out that substantial direct extrarectal spread is more reliably detected on a CT scan than is nodal involvement. It was recently my privilege to examine a Leeds surgeon, Paul Durdey, in his mastership thesis which was entirely devoted to the subject of pre-operative assessment, and he drew attention in this to the importance of combining CT scanning with CEA investigations to determine the locally advanced tumour. With the rise in the use of radiotherapy for such tumours, this pre-operative assessment may become increasingly important in future.

The second point that the Guildford group made in *The Lancet* interests me very greatly. It related to the total failure of their group to reproduce the figures formerly published by Quirke and Norman Williams and their associates from Leeds which suggested that lateral margin involvement was a reliable predicter of clinical local recurrence during the early years of follow-up. The Guildford group found this test quite useless, with only 1 of 13 local recurrences being thus predicted, and only 1 out of 12 involved lateral margins going on to develop local recurrence. The explanation for this is very interesting indeed, and it reflects the extremely slow rate of growth of this particular tumour. The Leeds specimens were from a range of surgeons delivering a local recurrence rate of around 30% within 18 months. The Guildford specimens on the other hand came from our own Chris Marks who was delivering a local recurrence rate of 7%. My presumption is therefore that the mesorectal edges of Chris's specimens approximated more nearly to the true peripheral margin of the visceral mesentery. Interestingly, therefore, when one of the Guildford specimens had involved edges, the patient's fate was already sealed because all such patients died with metastases before they had time to develop the local recurrence. One can thus say that mesorectal edge or lateral margin involvement is a predictor of preventable local recurrence in most cases, and indeed comparison of these two series confirms my own theory that the totality of the removal of the visceral mesentery is indeed the major predictor of local recurrence.

Ideas for the Future

The precise detail of the local clearance of a rectal carcinoma is clearly of major importance. There are therefore challenges to improve the teaching and understanding of the anatomy of the deeper part of the pelvis. High-grade high-definition interactive video teaching systems for surgeons seem a possible way forward. Pre-operative imaging may also be important in planning the surgery and also in deciding which cases require pre-operative radiotherapy. The higher the quality of the surgery the lower will be the number of patients who require this adjuvant modality.

Therapy of the Primary Tumour

P.F. SCHOFIELD

The treatment options for carcinoma of the rectum have expanded in recent years. In order to improve treatment, we must consider the means of spread of the tumour and the causes of treatment failure. In general, treatment failure may be classified into distant recurrence or local recurrence, and in some patients both occur. The realisation of the importance of distant metastases has led to adjuvant therapy directed towards the liver by chemotherapy delivered by the portal vein [1] or a systemic route [2]. Further, there has been an increasing awareness that monitoring for hepatic metastases by intraoperative ultrasound may identify operable lesions in the liver [3].

In the main, I want to concentrate here on the range of therapies used to treat the primary tumour. There is certainly some evidence that peri-operative radiotherapy as an adjuvant to surgery will reduce the local recurrence rates [4]. Tumour aggressiveness varies widely, so tumours with low-grade malignant potential can, in theory, be adequately treated by a relatively local procedure, whilst highly malignant tumours may well be incurable by any modality available at present. In my practice, a quarter to a third of the patients who present for surgery have metastatic disease already, and operations in this group can only be for palliation. The remaining patients represent a wide spectrum from small, low-grade malignant tumours to large, fixed growths. Of these operable tumours, a majority fall into the group that is suitable for radical resection, a topic which my colleague Mr. Heald has discussed. I intend to talk about the small number of patients who may be suitable for less radical procedures and the patients who may require supra-radical procedures.

The Small Rectal Cancer

It is now generally agreed that cancer developing in a polyp without involvement of the stalk can be treated satisfactorily by local excision. Small rectal tumours which have not penetrated through the full thickness of the wall (Dukes A) are unlikely to have metastasised even to lymph nodes, and these patients would also appear to be suitable for local treatment provided we can assess the degree of involvement accurately. In experienced hands, rectal examination under anaesthetic gives a lot of information, and recently intrarectal ultrasound has increased the accuracy of assessment [5]. We select patients for local treatment if they are shown by palpation and ultrasound to have small tumours entirely confined to the rectal wall with no demonstrable lymph node metastases. Local excision [6], local diathermy destruction [7] or resection [8], contact radiotherapy [9] or interstitial implant radiotherapy [10] have all produced good results in carefully selected tumours. These patients should be closely followed so that if the local treatment fails they can be "salvaged" by radical surgery.

The Large Fixed Tumour

In this group of patients, preliminary assessment by examination under an anaesthetic, pelvic CT or NMR is essential. Intrarectal ultrasound is also useful when it is possible, but on some occasions the tumour is so bulky that this examination is difficult. It is important to assess the involvement of other organs. Particularly in males, a low rectal tumour may involve the prostate and a rather higher tumour may involve the bladder base. In either of these situations, one has to consider the possibility of total pelvic clearance [11]. It is important, before advising this radical procedure, to exclude metastatic disease, so adequate imaging of both the liver and lungs must be performed. With these bulky tumours we believe that moderately high dosage pre-operative radiotherapy is desirable with surgery delayed for 6–8 weeks [12].

Turning to the surgery, if the urinary tract is involved, it may be necessary to carry out a total pelvic clearance in order to achieve adequate tumour excision. In low tumours it is rarely possible to do a restorative resection, but in tumours which are highly placed, this can be done despite the radiotherapy. After mobilising the colon we have found it possible to detach a loop of distal colon and use this as the urinary conduit, transplanting the ureters into the proximal end and bringing the distal end out in the right iliac fossa. The intact residual colon can always be adequately mobilised to effect a colorectal anastomosis or to fashion a left iliac fossa colostomy, as appropriate. In females, the urinary tract is usually protected by the uterus and vagina, but it is desirable to know about involvement of the genital tract as a posterior pelvic clearance may be indicated. It may be necessary to remove most of the vagina with the uterus and rectum but a detached loop of colon can easily be used to construct a neo-vagina [13].

Conclusion

We have many treatment options available for patients with carcinoma of the rectum. It is important to realise that rectal tumours have a wide spectrum of behaviour. Some remain localised and have a low tendency to metastasise but some metastasise very early. Our management should be personalised to the individual patient and can range from local peranal treatment to total pelvic clearance, depending on the assessment of the situation. The position of adjuvant radiotherapy or chemotherapy is still not fully resolved, but the appropriate surgical treatment and the tumour biology appear to be the most important aspects in determining outcome.

Hepatic Metastases

J. PETTAVEL

At initial laparotomy, 15%–20% of patients operated on for cancer of the rectum are found to harbour hepatic metastases. 15%–20% more patients will later demonstrate hepatic metastases during the follow-up period.

Early diagnosis of hepatic metastases has benefited from the progress made in radiologic imaging (CT, angio-CT, isotopic emission tomography, immuno-scintigraphy) and from technological advances of the less expensive ultrasonography. Development of tumour markers is rapidly progressing, and the use of new monoclonal antibodies is opening new avenues in the diagnosis of rectal malignancies and their metastases.

For the time being, only surgery is able to cure patients with hepatic metastases, although one may, like Steele and Ravikumar [14], wonder if the good results of surgery do not reflect the selection of a small group of patients with less aggressive tumours. The conditions for successful surgery of liver secondaries were studied in the International Registry of Hepatic Metastases and published by Hughes, Scheele and Sugarbaker [15]. The number of metastases and the size of the free margin around the resected metastases are critical factors. A 5-year survival rate of 35% may be obtained after resection of single or two hepatic metastases, but the rate falls to 9% if three or four metastases are to be resected. A tumour-free margin of 1.0 cm allows a 5-year survival rate of 44%, but if the margin is less than 1.0 cm or if the margin is involved, survival falls to 20%. A survival rate of 32% may be obtained if metastases are located in the liver only, but if cancer cells are found in the portal nodes, it falls to 4%. Clear surgical indications are relatively rare and, finally, only 5% of these patients may survive for 5 or 10 years. Hepatic metastases are too often bilateral and multiple, precluding surgical resection. Moreover, extrahepatic metastases, if not already present at the time of diagnosis of the hepatic secondaries, may develop later. Adson [16] recently presented an excellent synthesis of prognostic factors.

Chemotherapy has practically never cured any patient of hepatic metastases. Regional chemotherapy (hepatic artery infusion) may give complete or partial temporary remission in more than 50% of cases, but that an objective increase in survival time occurs has been denied by most authors until recently. Chang et al. [17], amongst others, have now demonstrated statistically significant increases in the duration of survival for patients free of extrahepatic metastases.

For the last 25 years, it has been doubtful whether arterial chemotherapy was better than systemic chemotherapy for the treatment of hepatic secondaries. We know now, thanks to the randomized studies of Kemeny et al. [18], Chang et al. [17] and Hohn et al. [19], that the results of hepatic artery infusion are certainly better than those of systemic or portal intravenous infusion. This increase of remission rate is statistically significant (Table 1).

The combination of 5-fluorouracil and Levamisole was used successfully in adjuvant studies, but results on the treatment of advanced cancer are still not available.

It is impossible to compare results of different treatments if the series that are studied are not really comparable. This may seem obvious, but was completely forgotten by most authors until recently. We have presented the different classifications of hepatic metastases since 1966 [20]. Our classification was simple, based on the number and size of metastases and level of alkaline phosphatase. Results were reproducible and survival prognosis could be thus ascertained. A few years ago we proposed a more comprehensive classification that gave birth to the international staging system presented by Van de Velde and Sugarbaker [21]. Gennari et al. [22] built up a more complicated classification, and Gennari told us recently that he had an excellent prognostic correlation. No matter what classification is used, it is urgent that one be generally adopted.

For the last 25 years, we have been using the same drugs: 5-fluorouracil and 5-FUDR; the use of mitomycin C does not seem to have really improved the results. Recently, cisplatin and Adriamycin combinations have been said to be helpful, but these represent only second-line treatment. The use of murine monoclonal antibodies has permitted extremely interesting progress in the diagnosis of primary and metastatic tumours of colorectal origin. Adding ^{131}I to the antibody allows therapeutic use, but our first results, as reported by Mach et al. [23], as well as those of the few other teams interested in this question, have not shown real clinical success. The use of chimeric antibodies gave us new hope quite recently. The ultimate goal is to use pure human antibodies but this has not been possible so far. It will permit repeated injections of therapeutic isotopic doses as well as

Table 1. Randomized studies showing statistically significant advantage of intra-arterial over intravenous infusions

	No. of patients		Objective remission (50% at CT)		Survival		Median time to progression (days)	
	i.a.	i.v.	i.a.	i.v.	i.a.	i.v.	i.a.	i.v.
N. Kemeny et al., Memorial Center, NY 1987	48	45	50% (24)	20% (10)	(median, months) 17	12		
			$p < 0.001$					
A. Chang et al., Natl. Cancer Inst., 1987	21	29	62% (13)	17% (5)	(2 years) 47%	13%		
			$p < 0.003$		$p < 0.03$			
D. Hohn, Univ. San Francisco, 1987	51	59	37% (19)	10% (6)			658	203
			$p < 0.002$				$p < 0.0003$	

more selective fixation onto the tumour cells. We think that the future may lie in the combined use of "hot" monoclonal antibodies and arterial chemo-infusion.

For the moment, the problem of chemotherapeutic toxicity remains unsolved. Toxicity with the intravenous route of administration of drugs is double: hematopoietic and digestive. Hematopoietic toxicity rarely necessitates the interruption of treatment, but intractable diarrhoea due to continuous infusion of fluorinated pyrimidines often results in having to discontinue treatment. The toxicity of hepatic arterial infusion is different. The so-called chemical hepatitis is rather benign and transitory, almost always disappearing rapidly after discontinuation of treatment. Gastroduodenal ulceration is reported in all series, but experienced surgeons now know that a more careful dissection of the hepatic artery prevents the appearence of this unpleasant complication. If a duodenal ulcer is nevertheless demonstrated, discontinuing the treatment is mandatory and surgical exploration is mostly always helpful. Minute arteries originating from the main trunk of the hepatic artery are then ligated and the ulcers always immediately heal. The most troublesome side effect of hepatic artery infusion is biliary toxicity. Simple knowledge of anatomy explains quite well why this biliary toxicity is more important next to the bifurcation of the main biliary ducts and at the level of the gallbladder (Fig. 1).

The concentration of the toxic drug is higher in the small arteries supplying peribiliary vascular plexuses and the surrounding tissues at the origin of the main bile ducts. We have observed obliteration of small arterial vessels in this region, as well as ischaemic necrosis of the mucosa of the bile ducts, and permeation of bile through the duct wall, resulting in necrosis of the bile ducts and intense fibrous reaction around them. The final stage of this process may result in complete obliteration of the main bile ducts. We have reported the succession of toxic side effects elsewhere [24].

The studies of Roemeling, Hrushevski and colleagues [25, 26], as well as the research of Levi et al. [27], have convinced us of the importance of chronotherapy. Toxicity of all drugs seems to differ depending on time of administration. There is a sort of "free window" of toxicity somewhere in the 24 h, which is specific for each drug. Since we moved from constant-rate infusions to time-qualified infusions of 5-FUDR using the completely implanted and programmable Synchroned Medtronic Pump, we have been surprised to note that the level of alkaline phosphatase and the level of transaminase return to normal if they were abnormal at the beginning of treatment. If the level of these enzymes was normal at the beginning of treatment they never increased to more than double the baseline level, and then only for a short time. This is completely different from what we were accustomed to observe with constant rate infusions with Infusaid 400 pumps.

Chronotherapy may be administered by vascular access ports of many available types or by completely implanted pumps. Pumps are said to cost a lot more money than simple access ports. This is true if only the catalogue

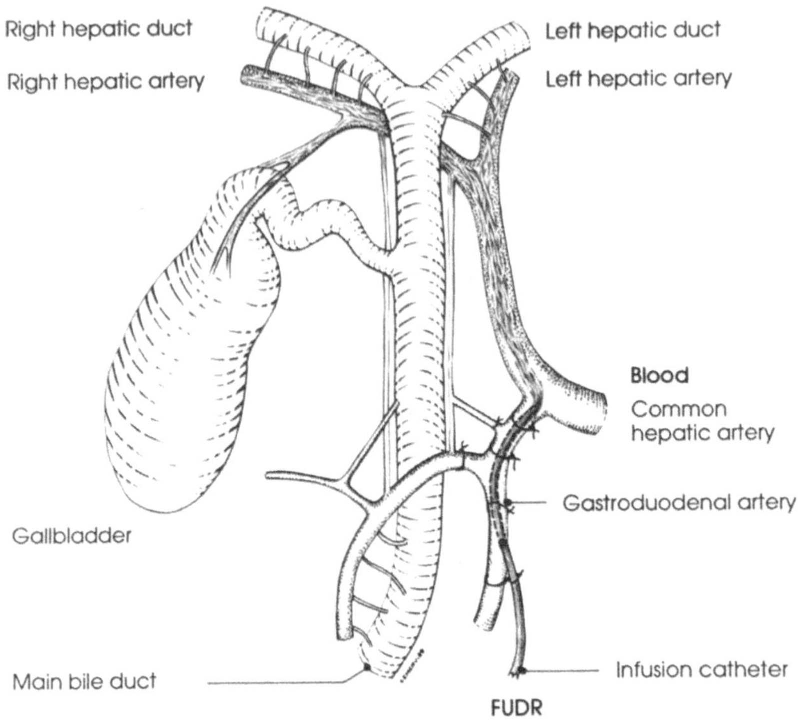

Fig. 1. Anatomical distribution of arterial branches explains high drug concentrations and high toxicity near the biliary duct bifurcation

price of the device is considered, but becomes wrong after less than 12 months of treatment, as shown by Elias and Rougier [28]. When one thinks that complications are more numerous with access ports than with implanted pumps, one may say that the future belongs to implantable programmable pumps. Elias et al. [29] also demonstrated that the presence of two separate hepatic arteries did not preclude the use of only one catheter as long as the second artery was ligated. Our own experience confirms entirely the experience of the French authors.

In conclusion, one may say that patients presenting with hepatic metastases of colorectal origin cannot be cured for the moment by treatment other than surgical resection of the metastases. When this is impossible due to the number of metastatic deposits, hepatic artery infusion can offer partial or complete temporary remissions to more than 50% of patients. These remissions do not seem to influence survival time, except in those patients who are free of all extrahepatic metastases. Time-qualified infusions using programmable implanted pumps are, in our opinion, the best available treatment if surgery is impossible. The future may show that benefits will be obtained by the joint use of new "hot" monoclonal antibodies and regional chemotherapy.

Adjuvant Radiotherapy

R.O. MIRIMANOFF

Although recent studies have clearly demonstrated the efficacy of adjuvant radiotherapy given after, before or during surgery for locally advanced rectal cancer, its exact role is not always well defined. In order to clarify certain issues, several pertinent questions should be adressed with regard to radiotherapy in rectal cancer:

1. Does local adjuvant therapy makes sense?
2. Does radiotherapy work as a local treatment?
3. Are there any suggestions that adjuvant radiotherapy works?
4. Is there proof that adjuvant radiotherapy works?
5. Has adjuvant radiotherapy any impact on survival?
6. What are the respective advantages of preoperative and postoperative radiotherapy?
7. What is the risk of long-term complications after adjuvant radio-therapy?
8. How can the risk of small bowel complications be reduced?
9. What can be done in locally advanced Rectal Cancer?
10. What are the future research directions?

The purpose of this presentation is to try at least partially to answer these questions by reviewing the pertinent available literature.

Does Local Adjuvant Therapy Make Sense?

In order to determine whether some sort of adjuvant therapy, including radiation therapy, is needed or not, it is necessary to determine the pattern and risk of failure with respect to various tumour parameters.

Table 2 shows the risk of local failure from five American surgical series [31–35] as a function of the Gunderson–Sosin staging system [30]. From these studies, it is evident that the risk of local failure increases both with the degree of rectal wall invasion by the tumor and with the presence of metastatic lymph nodes. Of all failures, local failure alone represents between 50% and 70%. The risk reaches significant values beyond Gunderson stage B2, and the majority of patients with C2–C3 lesions will suffer from a local recurrence. Thus, according to these data, adjuvant therapy makes sense and is needed in Gunderson–Sosin stage B2 and beyond.

Table 2. Rate of local failure as a function of the Gunderson–Sosin [30] staging system in surgical series

Series	No. of patients	Year	Local failure (%) according to stage							
			A	B_1	B_2	B_3	C_1	C_2	C_3	Ref.
Maine	107	1977	0	17	51[a]		20	78[b]		31
MGH	142	1983	–	8	23	53	50	47	67	32
University of Florida	280	1976	0	15	19	34	–	21	52	33
Brigham Hospital	281	1980	–	–	33[a]		35[c]		50	34
Memorial	412	1984	0	14	30[a]		23[c]		49	35

[a] B_2 plus B_3
[b] C_2 plus C_3
[c] C_1 plus C_2

Table 3. Rate of local failures as a function of the Gunderson–Sosin staging system in retrospective postoperative radiation therapy series

Series	No. of patients	Local failure (%) according to stage							
		A	B_1	B_2	B_3	C_1	C_2	C_3	Ref.
Jefferson	31	–	–	–	6	–	–	–	38
MDAH	105	–	0	4	31	8	18	20	39
MGH	165	–	0	9	0	20	21	53	40
Mayo	139	–	–	18	33	10	26	14	41

Does Radiation Therapy Work as an Anticancer Treatment in Rectal Adenocarcinoma?

For many years, gastrointestinal adenocarcinoma were considered "radioresistant" and irradiation of these tumors was contra-indicated. This was derived, however, from older studies, employing radiotherapy methods which were primitive by today's standards. For many technical and physical reasons efficient treatment could not be delivered to deep-seated lesions without causing unacceptable complications. Almost 30 years ago, Wang and Schultz at the Massachusetts General Hospital, using high-energy photon beams, showed that radiotherapy of inoperable cancer could be delivered safely, that the symptomatic response rate was above 80%, and that 5% of these patients unexpectidly survived 5 years [36]. Fifteen years ago, Papillon published his technique of intracavitary radiotherapy for noninfiltrative rectal cancer in elderly patients. Local control – or definitive tumor destruction – was obtained in over 90% of cases and the 5-year survival reached about 80% [37]. These two pioneering works were followed by many others demonstrating that, contrary to previous opinion, radiotherapy is an effective anticancer agent in rectal cancer.

Table 4. Rate of local failures in retrospective preoperative radiation therapy series

Series	No. of patients	Local failures (%)	Ref.
Combes	344	8	42
EORTC*	121	15	43
Rochester	64	9	44
St Louis	112	2	45

* prospective study

Table 5. Rates of local failures in postoperative radiotherapy randomised trials

Series	No. of patients	Decrease in local failure (%)	*p*	Ref.
GTSG	227	25% → 16%	0.06	47
Denmark	494	22% → 25%	NS	46
NSABP	555	24% → 16%	0.06	48
MRC III	412	42 → 14[a]	<0.001	49

[a] Actual number of recurrences

Are There any Suggestions that Adjuvant Radiotherapy Works?

Table 3 shows the results of four recently published retrospective studies of postoperative radiotherapy of rectal cancer [38–41]. As can be seen, the local failure rate as a function of the Gunderson–Sosin staging system [30] is relatively low except for stages C2–C3, and compares favourably with the pure surgical series. Table 4 shows the local failure rate of four preoperative radiation series [42–45]. Since therapy was given prior to surgery, staging could not be adequately assessed. However, the overall local failure rate is strikingly low and is in favour of a positive effect of radiotherapy. Thus, we can state that preoperative and postoperative data, when compared to surgical data, strongly suggest but do not prove that radiotherapy is an efficient adjuvant treatment in rectal cancer.

Is There Proof that Adjuvant Radiotherapy Works?

In order to demonstrate scientifically whether ionizing radiation is effective in rectal cancer, numerous projective randomized trials have been designed, eight of which are presented here.

Table 5 summarizes four large postoperative radiotherapy randomized trials from Europe and the United States. While the Danish study did not

Table 6. Results of preoperative radiotherapy trials

Series	No. of patients	Results	p	Ref.
MRC I	824	Downstaging	0.006	49
V.A.	361	Downstaging	0.001	50
MRC II	265	Increase in RFS	0.09	49
Brazil	68	Decrease in local failures	not computed	51

show any advantage of postoperative radiotherapy [46], the two American trials disclosed an improvement in local control of borderline statistical significance [46–48] and the early results of MRC III have demonstrated a net decrease ($p < 0.001$) in local failure in the radiotherapy group [49]. The four preoperative radiotherapy trials are shown in Table 6. In MRC II the recurrence-free survival is increased in the radiotherapy arm but the p value is only 0.09 [49]. In MRC I and the VA trial there was a statistically significant effect on downstaging ($p = 0.001$ to $p = 0.006$) in the adjuvant arm [49, 50]. From these studies, there is evidence that adjuvant pre- or postoperative radiotherapy has a positive impact on local disease.

Has Adjuvant Radiotherapy any Impact on Survival?

Of all randomized trials of pre- and postoperative radiotherapy [46–51], and including the preliminary results of one EORTC trial [52], none has shown that adjuvant local radiotherapy has a statistically significant impact on survival. However, in MRC II and III there is a trend ($p = 0.08$ and $p = 0.06$ respectively) towards an improved survival, which suggests that the apparent lack of effect in any of these studies might be due, at least in part, to a statistical type II error (risk of false-negative results because of an insufficient number of patients in each study arm). Another reason for the apparent absence of improved survival may be the similar rates of metastatic deaths in all treatment groups. Interestingly, patients included in the chemotherapy and radiotherapy arm of the GTSG study had a highly significant improvement in survival compared to no adjuvant therapy ($p = 0.01$) [47].

What Are the Respective Advantages of Pre- and Postoperative Radiotherapy?

Both approaches have been shown to decrease the local failure rate. In preoperative radiotherapy, the target is easier to identify by the radio-oncologist, there is no separation of anatomical planes and no subsequent risk of spreading the areas to be irradiated, and the delay between radiotherapy and surgery is kept to a minimum. Preoperative radiotherapy is the only alternative for advanced (fixed or tethered) tumours. In postoperative radiotherapy, the radio-oncologist has a better knowledge of the tumour stage and adequate information about the pathology, and can therefore make a more appropriate case selection.

What Is the Risk of Long-Term Complications After Adjuvant Radiotherapy?

In treating rectal cancers with doses of 45–55 Gy, the major complication risk is small bowel damage, perhaps resulting in fistulae or stenosis. In most series in which this complication was recorded, the small bowel complication rate was between 5% and 7% [40, 41, 43, 47, 53]. However, when large fields, poor techniques and concommitant chemotherapy were used, the risk could be as high as 11%–25% [43, 54]. With appropriate surgical and radiotherapy techniques, excluding part or all small bowel from the irradiation field [55], the complication rate should be kept below 5%.

How Can the Risk of Small Bowel Complications Be Reduced?

The most efficient way to avoid complications is to consider each patient prospectively and individually in a multidisciplinary approach, where the medical oncologist, radiation oncologist and surgeon evaluate the case together prior to any therapy. Surgical measures to remove the small bowel from the irradiated area are important. Techniques such as pelvic vicryl mesh slings [56] or other pelvic reconstruction techniques [55] should be used widely. Radiation oncology preventive measures include an exact individual knowledge of the position of organs at risk, sophisticated planning techniques, the use of megavoltage, isocentric units, and an appropriate selection of dose and fractionation [55, 57]. At MGH, the continuous use of these techniques has resulted in a complication rate of 4%, which is not superior to that of surgery alone [40, 53].

What Can Be Done in Locally Advanced Rectal Cancer?

Facing the problem of locally far-advanced lesions, corresponding clinically to tethered or to fixed lesions, many surgeons wonder if anything other than a palliative excision is worth trying. However, early experience at Tuffts [58] and MGH [59] indicated that preoperative moderate- to high-dose radiotherapy could change the situation well enough to make a curative resection feasible. Currently, several centres have initiated aggressive protocols for advanced tumours, including external beam preoperative radiotherapy, surgery, and intraoperative electron beam radiotherapy. At

MGH, Tepper et al. treated 75 patients with such an approach: patients presented either with far-advanced or recurrent rectal cancer [60]. In patients with primary advanced lesions, the 3-year survival was 58% and only three local failures were recorded [60]. Gunderson, at the Mayo Clinic, obtained a 4-year survival of 53% for primary advanced and 23% for recurrent tumours with a similar programme [61]. Calvo in Spain reported on his experience with 27 patients with a shorter follow-up of 11 months. The local control varied between 60% and 90% in the three groups of patients (recurrent disease after radiotherapy, without radiotherapy, or residual disease at surgery). From these rather preliminary data, one can say that new, sophisticated and agressive radiotherapeutic approaches used in conjonction with surgery represent promising ways to treat locally advanced rectal cancers.

What Are the Future Research Directions?

From the answers given to the nine previous questions, it is possible to conclude that there is a definitive and important role for radiotherapy in rectal cancers. In operable lesions, phase III studies should continue to assess the respective role of adjuvant pre- or postoperative radiotherapy and systemic therapy, using the concept of spatial cooperation [63]. In inoperable tumours, studies of preoperative radiotherapy, with or without chemotherapy, and surgery and intraoperative radiotherapy should continue, while in parallel other new modalities such as precision, high-dose conformation photon-beam therapy and particle radiotherapy should be further developed.

References

1. Metzger U (1988) Intraportal chemotherapy for colorectal hepatic metastases. Antibiot Chemother 40: 51–60
2. Buyse M, Zeleniuch-Jacquotte A, Chalmers TC (1988) Adjuvant therapy of colorectal cancer. JAMA 259: 3571–3578
3. Machi J et al (1987) Intraoperative ultrasonography in screening for liver metastases from colorectal cancer – comparative accuracy with traditional procedures. Surgery 101: 678–684
4. Jones DJ et al (1989) Predicting local recurrence of carcinoma of the rectum after pre-operative radiotherapy and surgery. Br J Surg 76: 1072–1075
5. Beynon J et al (1986) Endoluminal ultrasound in the assessment of local invasion in rectal cancer. Br J Surg 73: 474–477
6. Morson BC, Bussey HRJ, Samourian S (1977) Policy of local excision for early cancer of the rectum. Gut 18: 1045–1050
7. Crile G, Turnbull RB (1972) The role of electrocoagulation in the treatment of carcinoma of the rectum. Surg Gynecol Obstet 135: 391–396
8. Berry AR et al (1990) Endoscopic transanal resection of rectal tumours — a preliminary report of its use. Br J Surg 77: 134–137

9. Papillon J (1987) Resectable rectal cancers. Treatment by curative endocavity radiation. JAMA 231: 1385–1387
10. Schofield PF (1990) In: Caird FT, Brewin T (eds) Cancer in the elderly. Butterworth, Guildford, pp 124–135
11. Lopez MJ et al (1987) Exenterative surgery for locally advanced rectosigmoid cancers – is it worthwhile? Surgery 102: 644–651
12. James RD, Schofield PF (1985) Resection of "inoperable" rectal cancer following radiotherapy. Br J Surg 72: 279–281
13. Schofield PF, Barnard RJ, Tindall VR (1989) Surgical treatment of carcinoma involving the vagina. Br J Surg 76: 816–817
14. Steele G Jr, Ravikumar TS (1989) Resection of hepatic metastases from colorectal cancer. Ann Surg 210: 127–128
15. Hughes K, Scheele J, Sugarbaker PH (1989) Surgery for colorectal cancer metastatic to the liver. Surg Clin North Am 69: 339–359
16. Adson MA (1987) Resection of Liver metastases. When is it worthwhile? World J Surg 11: 511–520
17. Chang AE, Schneider PD, Sugarbaker PH, Simpson C, Culnane M, Steinberg SM (1987) A prospective randomized trial of regional versus systemic continuous 5-fluorodeoxyuridine chemotherapy in the treatment of colorectal liver metastases. Ann Surg 206: 685–693
18. Kemeny N, Daly J, Reichmann B, Geller N, Botet J, Oderman P (1987) Intrahepatic or systemic infusion of fluorodeoxyuridine in patients with liver metastases from colorectal carcinoma. Ann Int Med 107: 459–465
19. Hohn D, Stagg R, Friedman M, Ignoffu R, Hannigan J, Rayner A, Ignoffo J, Acord P, Lewis B (1989) A randomized trial of continuous intravenous versus hepatic intra-arterial floxuridine in patients with colorectal cancer metastatic to the liver: the Northern California oncology group trial. J Clin Oncol 7: 1646–1654
20. Pettavel J, Leyvraz S, Douglas P (1984) The necessity for staging liver metastases and standardizing treatment-response criteria. In: Van de Velde CJ, Sugarbaker PH (eds) Liver metastasis. Nijnhoff, Boston, pp 154–168
21. Van de Velde CJH, Veenhof CHN, Sugarbaker PH (1984) Methodology in the clinical study of liver metastases. In: Van de Velde CJH and Sugarbaker PH (eds) Liver metastasis. Nijnhoff, Boston, pp 358–373
22. Gennari L, Doci R, Bozzetti F, Veronesi V (1982) Proposal for clinical classification of liver metastases. Tumori 68: 1443–1449
23. Mach JP, Buchegger F, Bischof-Delaloye A, Curchod S, Mosimann F, Givel JC, Pettavel J, Delaloye B (1988) Localization of radio-labelled monoclonal anti-CEA antibodies and fragments in colon carcinoma. Diagnostic and therapeutic approaches. In: Fourth congress of the European Society of Surgical Oncology, Paris, 1988, p 90 (abstract)
24. Pettavel J, Gardiol D, Bergier N, Schnyder P (1988) Necrosis of main bile ducts caused by hepatic artery infusion of FUDR. Reg Cancer Treat 2: 83–92
25. Roemeling RV, Hrushesky WJM (1987) Circadian shaping of FUDR infusion reduces toxicity even at high dose intensity. Proc ASCO 6: 44 (abstract 170)
26. Roemeling RV, Rabatin J, Tuchmann, Buchit K, Moore J, Hrushesky WJM (1988) Circadian timing and mode of Fluoropyrimidine Administration markedly impact organ-specific toxicity and maximal dose intensity. In: Third international conference of Chronopharmacology, Nice, abstract RT-5
27. Levi F, Boughattas NA, Blazsek (1988) Comparative murine chronotoxicity of anticancer agents and related mechanism. Annu Rev Chronopharmacol 4: 284–332
28. Elias D, Rougier P, Bognel C, Ducreux M, Droz JP, Lumbroso J, Lasser P (1988) Intra-arterial chemotherapy for liver metastases from colorectal cancer. A comparison between implantable pump and subcutaneous access. Neth J Surg
29. Elias D, Lasser P, Rougier P (1987) A simplified surgical technical procedure for intra-arterial chemotherapy in secondary liver cancer. Experience in 50 patients. Eur J Surg Oncol 13: 441–448

30. Gunderson LL, Sosin H (1974) Arias of failure found at reoperation (second or symptomatic look) following "curative surgery" for adenocarcinoma of the rectum. Cancer 34: 1278–1292
31. Gilbert SG (1977) The case for adjuvant radiotherapy in adenocarcinoma of the rectum. J Maine Med Ass 68: 355–359
32. Rich T, Gunderson LL, Lew R et al (1983) Patterns of recurrence of rectal cancer after potentially curative surgery. Cancer 52: 1317–1329
33. Cass AW, Million RR, Pfaff WW (1976) Patterns of recurrence following surgery alone for adenocarcinoma of the colon and rectum. Cancer 37: 2861–2865
34. Olsen RM, Perencevich NP, Malcolm AW et al (1980) Patterns of recurrence following curative resection of adenocarcinoma of the colon and rectum. Cancer 45: 2969–2974
35. Pilipshen SJ, Heilweil M, Quan SH (1989) Patterns of pelvis recurrence following definitive resection of rectal cancer. Cancer 53: 1354–1362
36. Wang CC, Schulz MD (1962) The role of radiation therapy in the management of carcinoma of the sigmoid, rectosigmoid and rectum. Radiology 79: 1–5
37. Papillon J (1975) Intracavitary irradiation of early rectal cancer for cure: a series of 186 cases. Cancer 36: 696–701
38. Mohiuddin M, Marks G, Kramer S, Pajak T (1984) Adjuvant radiation therapy for rectal cancer. Int J Radiation Oncol Biol Phys 10: 997–980
39. Vigliotti A, Rich TA, Romsdahl MM et al (1987) Postoperative adjuvant radiotherapy for adenocarcinoma of the rectum and rectosigmoid. Int J Radiation Oncol Biol Phys 13: 999–1006
40. Tepper JD, Cohen AM, Wood WC et al (1987) Postoperative radiation therapy of rectal cancer. Int J Radiation Oncol Biol Phys 13: 5–10
41. Schild SE, Martenson JA, Gunderson LL et al (1989) Postoperative adjuvant therapy of rectal cancer: an analysis of disease control, survival and prognostic factors. Int J Radiation Oncol Biol Phys 17: 55–62
42. Combes PF, Gary-Bobo J, Naja A (1983) Câncers du rectum: radiothérapie préopératoire (344 cas). Bull Cancer 70: 317–322
43. Boulis-Wassif S, Gerard A, Loygue J (1984) Final results of a randomized trial on the treatment of rectal cancer with preoperative radiotherapy alone or in combination with 5-fluorouracil, followed by radical surgery. Cancer 53: 1811–1818
44. Haghbin, Sischy B, Hinson J (1988) Combined modality preoperative therapy in poor prognostic rectal adenocarcinoma. Radiother Oncol 13: 75–81
45. Roe JP, Kodner IJ, Walz B, Fry R (1982) Preoperative radiation therapy for rectal carcinoma. Dis Colon Rectum 25: 471–473
46. Balslev I, Pedersen M, Teglbjaerg PS et al (1986) Postoperative radiotherapy in Dukes B and C carcinoma of the rectum and rectosigmoid. Cancer 58: 22–28
47. Thomas PRM, Lindblad AS (1988) Adjuvant postoperative radiotherapy and chemotherapy in rectal carcinoma: a review of the Gastrointestinal Tumor Study Group experience. Radiother Oncol 13: 245–252
48. Fisher B, Wolmark N, Rockette H et al (1988) Postoperative adjuvant chemotherapy or radiotherapy for rectal cancer: results from NSABP protocol R-01. J Nat Cancer Inst 80: 21–29
49. Hardcastle JD (1989) Results of medical research council adjuvant radiotherapy trials in the treatment of rectal cancer. EORTC symposium on advances in gastrointestinal tract cancer research and treatment (abstract)
50. Higgins G, Humphrey EW, Dwight RW et al (1986) Preoperative radiation and surgery for cancer of the rectum. VASOG trial II. Cancer 58: 352–359
51. Neto JAR, Quilici FA, Reis JA (1989) A comparison of non-operative vs preoperative radiotherapy in rectal carcinoma. Dis Colon Rectum 32: 702–710
52. Nordlinger B, Buyse M, Pene F et al (1989) Postoperative radiotherapy in rectal carcinoma: EORTC trial. EORTC symposium on advances in gastrointestinal tract cancer research and treatment (abstract)

53. Hoskins G, Gunderson LL, Dosoretz D, Galdabini J (1980) Adjuvant postoperative radiotherapy in carcinoma of the rectum and rectosigmoid. Int J Radiation Oncol Biol Phys 6: 1379–1380
54. Withers HR, Romsdahl MM (1977) Postoperative radiotherapy for adenocarcinoma of the rectum and rectosigmoid. Int J Radiation Oncol Biol Phys 2: 1069–1074
55. Gunderson LL, Russel AH, Llewllyn HJ et al (1985) Treatment planning for colorectal cancer: radiation and surgical techniques and value of small bowel films. Int J Radiation Oncol Biol Phys 11: 1379–1393
56. Deutsch AA, Stern HS (1989) Technique of insertion of pelvic vicryl mesh sling to avoid postradiation enteritis. Dis Colon Rectum 32: 628–630
57. Tepper JE (1983) Radiation therapy of colorectal cancer. Cancer 51: 2528–2534
58. Emami B, Pilepich M, Willet C et al (1982) Effect of preoperative irradiation on resectability of colorectal carcinomas. Int J Radiation Oncol Biol Phys 8: 1295–1299
59. Dosoretz PJ, Gunderson LL, Hedberg S et al (1983) Preoperative irradiation for unresectable rectal and rectosigmoid carcinomas. Cancer 52: 814–818
60. Tepper JE, Wood WC, Cohen AM (1989) Treatment of locally advanced rectal cancer with external beam radiation, surgical resection, and intraoperative radiation terapy. Int J Radiation Oncol Biol Phys 16: 1437–1444
61. Gunderson LL, Martin K, Beart RW et al (1988) Intraoperative and external beam irradiation for locally advanced rectal cancer. Ann Surg 207: 52–59
62. Calvo FE, Algarra SM, Azinovic I et al (1989) Intraoperative radiotherapy for recurrent and/or residual colorectal cancer. Radiother Oncol 15: 135–140
63. Tubiana M, Arriagada R, Cosset JM (1985) Sequencing of drugs and radiation. Cancer 55: 2131–2139

Complex Fistula-in-Ano: Aetiology, Management and Functional Results

J.D. Hardcastle, M.-C. Marti, J.P.S. Thomson, R.H. Grace,
A. Akovbiantz, and P. Buchmann

What Is a Complex Anal Fistula and How Can These Lesions Be Classified?

J.D. Hardcastle

The successful treatment and understanding of fistula-in-ano requires knowledge of the anatomy of the anal canal, the pelvic musculature and the pathogenesis of fistula-in-ano. Sir Alan Parks made a number of contributions to our understanding of this problem, in the classification and pathogenesis of fistula-in-ano and in particular the importance of sepsis in the intersphincteric plane

Pathogenesis

The anal glands discharge through ducts at the mucocutaneous junction of the anal canal into the anal crypts. Glands are present in the intersphincteric plane and do not penetrate the external sphincter. Sepsis of the glandular elements is the cause of the primary abscess in the majority of cases of fistula-in-ano. An abscess in the intersphincteric plane can spread in both vertical or horizontal directions. Distal spread results in a perianal abscess at the anal margin, whereas upward spread results in an abscess within the rectal wall or in the supralevator space (Fig. 1). Horizontal spread may result in the infection discharging into the anal canal, usually at the site of the anal valves, or extension across the external sphincter and into the ischiorectal fossa. Infection in the intersphincteric, ischiorectal and pelvirectal spaces can spread circumferentially around the anal canal and rectum. This circumferential spread has in the past been referred to as "horseshoeing".

The classification of fistula-in-ano is based on the anatomy of the tracks in relation to the anal musculature and levator ani. Four main groups are recognised:

1. *Intersphincteric fistula* (Fig. 2). Intersphincteric fistulas spread in the plane between the internal and external sphincters. The most usual type

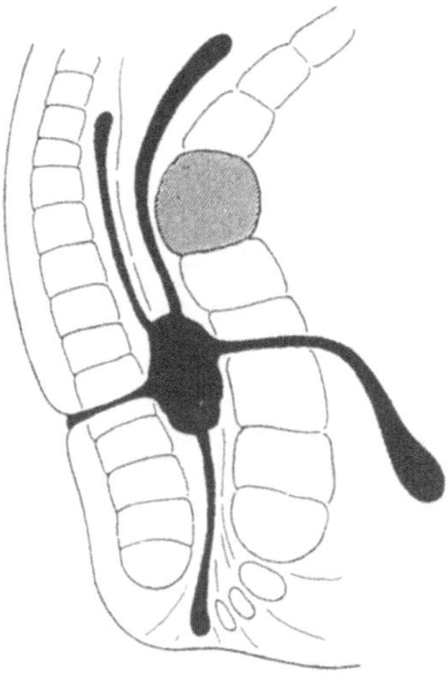

Fig. 1. Supralevator space. (From [20])

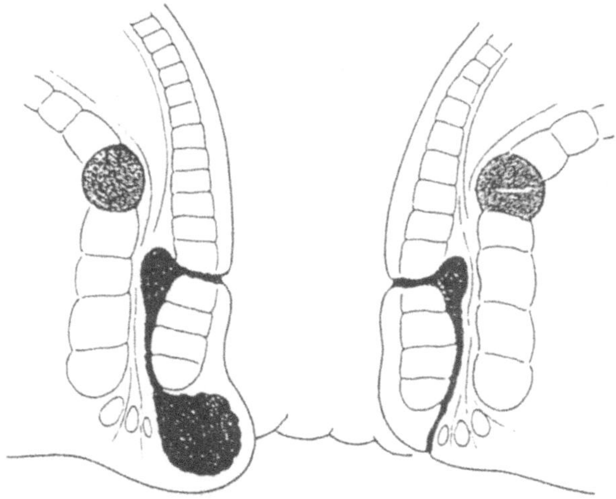

Fig. 2. Intersphincteric fistula. (From [20])

results when the intersphincteric abscess discharges near the anal margin as a perianal abscess. This type of fistula can easily be dealt with by laying open the abscess and fistula tracks into the anal canal.

2. *Trans-sphincteric fistula* (Fig. 3). In trans-sphincteric fistulas, infection passes from the intersphincteric plane, through the external sphincter and into the ischiorectal fossa, usually presenting as an ischiorectal abscess. The ischiorectal abscess may extend to the top of the ischiorectal fossa, resulting

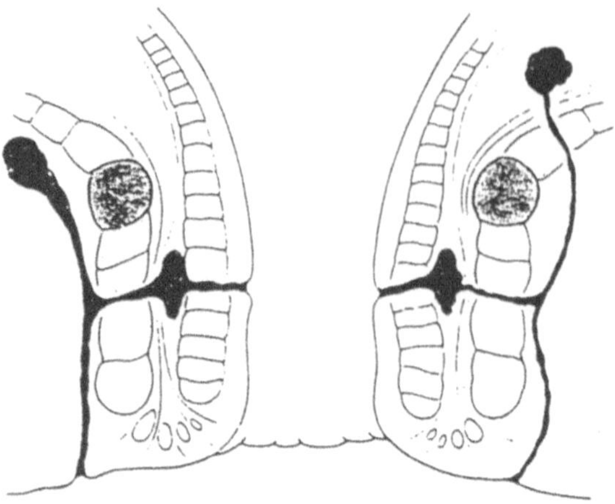

Fig. 3. Trans-sphincteric fistula. (From [20])

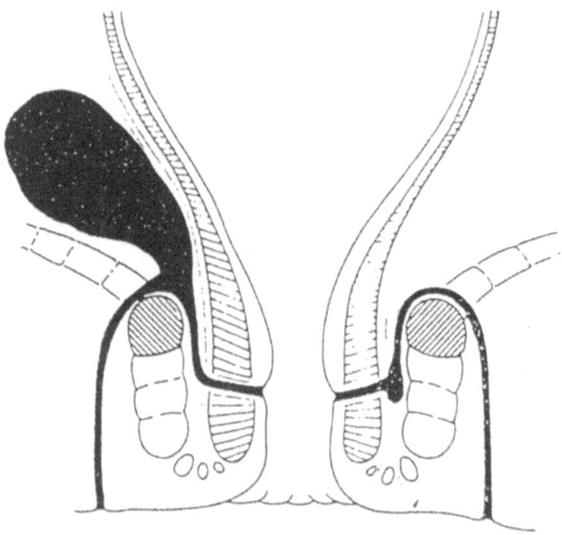

Fig. 4. Suprasphincteric fistula. (From [20])

in a blind track and in some cases the abscess may break through the levator muscle, resulting in a pelvic abscess. Usually the track passes through the external sphincter at a low level and can be safely laid open. Extension to the top of the ischiorectal fossa or through the levator muscles into the pelvic cavity may cause induration high in the anal canal. In these cases it is important to detect the site of the internal opening as the lower portion of the fistula can be safely laid open and the high tracks simply drained.

Fistulas with tracks passing through the upper portion of the external sphincter and puborectalis must be treated with caution.

3. *Suprasphincteric fistula* (Fig. 4). Suprasphincteric fistula results when a pelvic extension of an intersphincteric abscess discharges through the levator

ani into the ischiorectal fossa, the track passing over the puborectalis muscle. Fortunately, this type of fistula is very uncommon, and it is in these cases that a seton may be helpful in draining the high tracks, thereby preserving the upper part of the puborectalis.

4. *Extrasphincteric fistula.* Extrasphincteric fistulas pass entirely outside the sphincter muscles and are usually due to trauma or associated anorectal disease such as carcinoma, tuberculosis or Crohn's disease. A pelvic abscess draining through the perineum may also result in supersphincteric fistula if there is communication with the colon, the common causes are diverticular disease and Crohn's disease.

How May Complex Fistulas Be Diagnosed?

J.P.S. Thomson

The methods available for the assessment of fistula may be summarised as follows:

1. Palpation
2. Use of probes
3. Injection of the track
4. Lay open and use of curette
5. Imaging techniques
   - Fistulography
   - Anal ultrasonography
   - Computerised tomography
   - Magnetic resonance imaging

1. Palpation using a well-lubricated, gloved index finger is probably the best, and simplest method of identifying the type of fistula. The examination is feeling for the physical sign of induration. It may be possible to do this in the out-patient environment, but it is often best done under anaesthetic when much more information may be obtained.

2. Probes may be passed in the conscious patient but this may result in considerable discomfort. They are probably best used in the anaesthetised patient. For simple direct fistulae the passage of a probe from external to internal opening is straight-forward, but this is not the case with more complicated cases: indeed, it must always be remembered that there may not be an internal opening.

The types of probe are important, many being too large. The set of four Lockhart-Mummery fistula probes and a set of lacrimal probes are essential for this work, especially as some tracks may be very fine. To obtain the maximum value from these probes, it may be necessary to partially lay open the tracks first identified to discover subsequent ones.

3. Much has been said about injecting the track. Methylene blue may be used to stain granulation tissue, although it is usually easy to identify granulation tissue on the basis of its natural appearance, and to identify the internal opening. An alternative way of identifying the latter is by using a dilute solution of hydrogen peroxide, which should "bubble through" the opening.

4. When a track is laid open, the granulation tissue within it is clearly visible. This can then be removed using a curette, and the fibrous tissue underneath becomes visible. If granulation tissue cannot be removed with a curette, this strongly suggests there is a side track, and subsequent use of a probe may further determine the anatomy of the fistula.

5. Imaging techniques are being increasingly used to determine the pathoanatomy of fistulas. Fistulography with the injection of a contrast medium into the external opening has always been of value in determining the precise nature of extrasphincteric fistulas, especially those arising from disorders of the intestine within the pelvis, e.g. diverticular disease and Crohn's disease. This investigation does not, however, convey any more information than palpation in the other types of fistula.

Anal ultrasonography is currently being assessed as a diagnostic technique. In a preliminary study, Law et al. [1] indicated that it was useful in detecting complex fistulas, but more recently Seow and his colleagues [2] in a prospective trial have shown that digital examination is superior. Further evaluation is required as is evaluation of the much more expensive computerised tomography and magnetic resonance. It would seem though that the clinical method is supreme at the present.

Discussion

Grace: Why should one abscess drain intersphinctericically and the other one go across the external sphincter?

Thomson: Perhaps I could comment on the longitudinal muscle which has been so clearly shown using anal ultrasonography. It is a thick layer, and maybe it is the relationship of the primary intersphincteric abscess to that muscle which determines whether infection spreads in the intersphincteric space or whether it spreads across the external sphincter into the ischiorectal fossa.

Marti: There are over 12 anal glands but usually only one fistula or abscess. Why?

Thomson: Many are related to a previous fissure in the midline posteriorly.

Marti: How many people use methylene blue?
(Very few hands in the audience were raised.)

Hardcastle: I do not use methylene blue in every case, particularly when the internal opening is obvious. But if it is not immediately clear where the internal opening is, I find it helpful during the operation.

Buchmann: Methylene blue is also very useful for demonstrating side tracks.

Marti: I think it is very important not to overlook a side track, but you can also demonstrate it by insufflating air or by palpating without the need to disturb the tissue following injection of fluid.

Thomson: If you are using a curette, you will never curette the granulation tissue away from a side track. The persistence of granulation tissue leads you into the side track.

Marti: Who uses anal ultrasonography?

Mortensen: I strongly support the use of this investigation. The insufflation of air into the tracks may enhance the abnormality. I believe this is an investigation that should be done by the surgeon himself.

Hardcastle: I would agree. We have limited experience of this and there is a long learning curve. It took us a considerable time to learn the normal anatomy, let alone the abnormal. I am sure it ought to be the surgeon himself who does this examination, and it could be done well at the time of examination under anaesthetic.

Marti: Who performs fistulography? It is a frequent investigation in France. We only use it occasionally because it does not give exact data. It may be useful from time to time in complicated cases.

Buchmann: I would like to add a comment about fistulography. We rarely use it, but sometimes we use it after a small tube has been placed in the track to demonstrate an opening.

Marti: It is best to undertake fistulography yourself in association with the radiologist, as with ultrasonography.

What Is the Importance of Microbiological Investigation and How Is the Prognosis Affected by the Findings?

R.H. Grace

No surgeon can ignore aetiology when considering the management of any surgical problem. The anatomy of acute sepsis and fistula is well described, but it is microbiology that determines the correct management. Microbiology provides the data which will determine whether or not the surgeon will look for associated fistula disease when no fistula has been demonstrated at the initial acute drainage procedure. In this situation, the culture of bowel-derived organisms indicates the need for a second examination under anaesthetic (EUA) for a fistula-in-ano by an experienced surgeon. The culture of skin-derived organisms indicates that no second EUA is required, since the abscess is merely a "boil" which will not have originated as an intermuscular abscess, and, therefore, there will be no associated fistula. The evidence for these statements is well founded.

In 1973, a retrospective study [3] showed that while coliforms were the commonest organism to be cultured the incidence of *Staphylococcus aureus* was 16.9%. Previous [4, 5] and subsequent [6] studies confirmed this incidence as being between 15% and 28%. While accepting that sepsis will develop in the intermuscular space to produce an intersphincteric abscess [7–11], it was thought curious that such an abscess should grow *S. aureus* when this organism makes up such a small proportion of the faecal flora [12].

The evidence from the Wolverhampton (1) study [13] produced an explanation. The study was simple: 165 abscesses were examined under anaesthetic and drained. Pus (in a bottle) was sent for culture, and a fistula was sought. If none was found, a second EUA was performed 7–10 days later, and a fistula was again sought. A fistula found at either procedure was laid open. The surgeon had, by definition, no knowledge of the microbiology at the first EUA and he was deliberately not told the results of culture prior to the second EUA. The results were clear-cut; 62/114 (56.6%) patients whose pus grew bowel-derived organisms were found to have a fistula. In none of 34 patients with a skin-derived organism was a fistula demonstrated. Retrospective evidence however in a study published in the same year from St. Thomas' Hospital was not so clear-cut. While emphasising the importance of gut organisms, in particular bacteroides, fistulae were also found when skin-derived organisms had been demonstrated.

It was thought that the differences might reflect methodology. The Wolverhampton series was prospective, involving a single consultant surgeon with routine laboratory microbiology, whereas the St. Thomas' series relied on retrospective clinical data, involving numerous surgeons, mainly registrars, but had very detailed microbiology, with particular emphasis on anaerobes.

The surgical advantages of Wolverhampton were, therefore, combined with the microbiological expertise of St. Thomas' Hospital [15] – in a study now referred to as "The Pus in the Post". The method was as before. An EUA was performed and the abscess drained; a fistula was sought. The pus was posted to St. Thomas's Hospital. A second EUA was performed when no fistula had been demonstrated, and, as before, the surgeon had no knowledge of the results of microbiological tests. The microbiological studies paid particular attention to the bacteroids.

The results were again clear-cut. Eighty patients with anorectal sepsis were studied. All abscesses were drained, and pus was submitted for culture. If a fistula was found when the abscess was drained, it was laid open; otherwise a second examination under anaesthetic was performed within 7–10 days. In no case was sterile pus obtained. Gut aerobes, predominantly *Escherichia coli*, were isolated from 49 of 53 (92.5%) of patients with a fistula and 8 of 27 (29.6%) of those without ($p < 0.0001$). "Gut-specific bacteroids" predominantly *Bacteroides fragilis* were isolated from 47 of 53 (88.7%) patients with a fistula and 5 of 27 (18.5%) of those without ($p < 0.0001$). Anaerobes not specific to the gut, predominantly *B. asaccharolyticus*, *B. ureolyticus*, *Peptococci* and *Peptostreptococci*, in the absence of those specific to the gut, were isolated from 2 of 53 patients with a fistula (3.8%) and 17 of 27 (63%) of those without ($p < 0.0001$). *S. aureus* was isolated from only 1 of 53 (1.9%) patients with a fistula, but from 8 of 27 (29.6%) of those without ($p = 0.0012$).

The Wolverhampton (1) study concluded that the correct management of an acute anorectal abscess was EUA and drainage of pus with exploration for a fistula. A second EUA was required when no fistula was found initially, but culture grew bowel-derived organisms; a second procedure was not required when culture grew skin organisms. The Wolverhampton St. Thomas' study emphasised this, while clearly pointing out the separate significances of bowel- and skin-derived bacteroids.

All data however needed to be independently confirmed. This confirmation was supplied by Henrichsen and Christiansen [16] from Copenhagen in 1986. Their study was broadly similar except that they undertook fistulograms instead of a routine second EUA only performing this when a fistula was demonstrated. In their study no fistula-in-ano was demonstrated in any patient whose culture grew only skin-derived organisms; gut-derived organisms only were demonstrated in those patients with a fistula.

Correct management depends upon aetiology, and aetiology in anorectal sepsis is microbiology. The successful outcome of surgery requires the surgeon to take note of the microbiology while taking care of the sphincter. Unnecessary damage to the sphincter is unacceptable, and fistula surgery in acute anorectal sepsis is the province of an experienced surgeon. In practice, simple drainage in the acute phase followed by a second EUA by an experienced surgeon as dictated by microbiology is the safest management.

Marti: We must therefore ask our bacteriologist to check more accurately for the presence of the skin derived organisms and *Staphylococcus aureus*. This would avoid unnecessary surgical procedures in some patients.

Are Fistulas Complex from the Beginning or the Result of Poor Management?

Marti: I must express some concern about an unexperienced surgeon trying to find the fistula track at the initial procedure. I am also concerned about patients being treated with antibiotics for long periods of time before being referred for surgery. This might well result in a more complex situation arising.

Thomson: I am not sure that delay in treatment results in a more complex situation developing. Perianal abscesses will present promptly because of the pain produced by acute stretching of the perianal skin. However, a fistula developing in the fat of the ischiorectal fossa or the supralevator space is not likely to produce much in the way of symptoms until it has reached quite a large size. I would think that complexity is more likely to be due to natural pathogenesis than to poor management before referral for definitive surgery.

Hardcastle: I would support the last speaker, as it is very unusual to find a patient with a pure intersphincteric abscess. Infection has nearly always spread before presentation.

How Should Complex Fistulas Be Treated? Should There Be Only a Single Operative Procedure and How May Sphincter Integrity Be Preserved?

J.P.S. THOMSON

I am afraid that I do not have all the answers to the question of treatment of complex fistulas, which is probably one which has been discussed since the days of John of Arderne in the fourteenth century.

I really think we should abandon the term "complex fistula" and adhere to the classification Professor Hardcastle has already described, namely "intersphincteric, trans-sphincteric, suprasphincteric and extrasphincteric fistula". Probably 80% of fistulas are simple to manage and are either intersphincteric or low trans-sphincteric fistulas. Suprasphincteric and extrasphincteric fistulas are very rare, and so approximately 20% of fistulas will be trans-sphincteric fistulas with the primary track at or above the line of the anal valves, and these are potentially difficult to manage.

Each type of fistula should be considered individually when it comes to management. Most intersphincteric fistulas and trans-sphincteric fistulas where the internal opening is below the level of the line of the anal valves and which have a direct track can be simply laid open, healing will occur, and anal function will very largely be preserved intact. Others have discussed the possibility of excision of the track, coring-out the track, or the use of tight seton to cut through the muscle. Kronberg compared laying open with excision, and found that this resulted in a shorter healing time, but there was no difference in the recurrence rate after the two methods [17].

Trans-sphincteric fistulas with the primary track at or above the level of the line of the anal valves are the more difficult fistulas to treat. My policy is to lay open the intersphincteric space at the site of the primary infection and to drain the secondary tracks involving only division of the skin and adipose tissue. The question is what to do about the primary track; should it be divided or not? There is no doubt that division of the external sphincter leads to considerable deterioration in anal function and so surgeons are now trying to devise techniques to preserve external sphincter function: some use a seton as a drain, others as a muscle cutting device. Some advocate closing the internal opening with a sliding advancement flap (Dr Marti will tell us about these), and Mann and Clifton [18] have described a re-routing technique, to which Dr Buchmann will refer.

The late Sir Alan Parks used to make the point that the level at which the primary track crosses the external sphincter is not necessarily at the same height as the internal opening is within the anal canal – normally at the level of the line of the anal valves. Tracks may be lower, but more often they are higher and may pass between the external sphincter and puborectalis before entering the ischiorectal fossa.

May I describe the results of a series of patients published by Hugh Ross and myself in the *International Journal of Colorectal Diseases* in 1989 [19]. Thirty-four patients were described and a loose seton of monofilament nylon was used to drain the primary track. Healing was then allowed to occur round the seton which may take between 8 and 12 weeks. The seton was then removed, and in 44% of the patients healing occurred without division of the external sphincter; in the remainder the external sphincter had to be divided. There is a very considerable difference in the function between the two groups. Of the 15 patients in whom the sphincter was preserved, 12 were available for assessment with a follow-up of more than 1 year. Ten were fully continent (83%). Of those in whom the sphincter was divided, 16 were available for follow-up, but only 5 (32%) were fully continent. This difference is statistically significant. There were no recurrent fistulas in either group.

In the patients whose external sphincter was preserved, there were two patients who had impaired control of liquid faeces; however, in those in whom the external sphincter was divided ten were incontinent for liquid stool and eight for solid stool; five needed to wear a pad, and in three the sphincter function was so poor that a sphincter reconstruction was required.

Physiological studies have been done and, as one would expect, resting pressure and voluntary contraction in those in whom the external sphincter has been divided is considerably less than in those in whom it has been preserved.

What Is the Place of the Seton Drainage? Different Techniques and Methods of Our Own Method

P. BUCHMANN

Complex fistula-in-ano include high trans-sphincteric, suprasphincteric and extrasphincteric tracts as well as horseshoe fistulas. Because of the risk of a postoperative incontinence, laying open of fistula or a straight forward fistulectomy is not possible in these cases. Various ideas have been suggested including procedures needing a diverting colostomy. We shall concentrate on methods using a seton. Three different theories form the background for the use of a seton:

1. The progressively, tightened seton cuts through the sphincter muscles encircled by the fistula leaving a slowly progressing scare proximal to the tract ("traction élastique")
2. The seton helps in draining the wound and stimulates the formation of fibrous tissue. At a second operation the procedure is completed by dividing the residual track
3. The seton assists the closure of the internal fistula opening, making a second operation unnecessary

All three theories have their advocates.

"Traction Élastique"

A seton, usually of rubber, is used and tightened every 2–3 weeks, cutting the puborectalis sling and anal sphincter slowly as recommended by Arnous et al. [20a]. Others prefer a monofilament suture which has to be reknotted more frequently. Some surgeons increase traction by putting a weight on the sling but this is inconvenient for the patient. We have not used this method recently.

Multiple Stage Fistulectomy

When a deroofed abscess has healed apart from a clearly defined high fistula, various procedures have been recommended to heal the tract. Parks and Stitz advocate the use of a seton to produce a fibrous tissue reaction in order to fix the edges of the sphincter when divided. They claim a minimal risk of postoperative incontinence because retraction of the muscular fibres resulting in a large gap is prevented [21]. Some of our own recurrences after seton therapy were successfully treated by this method (see below).

Quite different is the rerouting procedure described by Mann and Clifton [18]. This procedure is summarized and instructively illustrated by

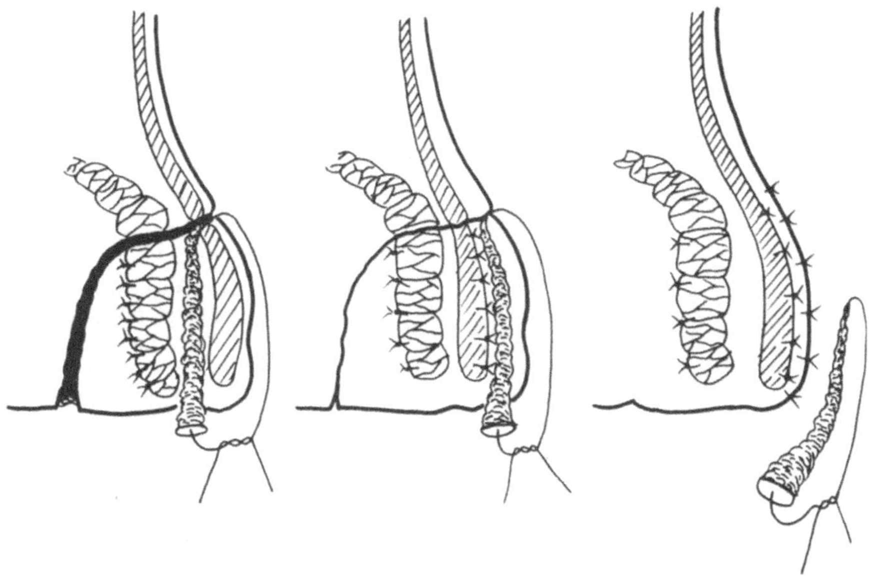

Fig. 5. Rerouting procedure described by Mann and Clifton. After seton drainage in a first operation the tract is moved of the intersphincteric space, in a second subcutaneously and in a third the fistula is excised [18]

Marti (Fig. 5) [22]. After healing of the wound the fibrotic tract with the seton is brought to the intersphincteric space by cutting and resuturing the external sphincter muscles. Then, 4–6 weeks later the tract is moved to the submucous plane by division and immediate repair of the internal sphincter. In a last step, the now submucosal fistula is removed and the wound closed. No deformation of the anal canal is left, resulting in a fully continent patient. This procedure is still new, and the complication rate is not yet known; we have no experience of it.

Seton Treatment Without Fistulectomy

In our department it is not our practice to treat a fistula during the deroofing of an abscess unless the tract is very obvious and low [23]. Probing at this stage is forbidden. Half of the abscesses will heal, the remaining half will have a fistula [24]. Treatment of the fistula is then by a second operation. We propose the following procedure for complicated fistulas (Fig. 6).

The infralevator of the extrasphincteric portion of the tract is excised by a conically shaped wound with the tip on the striated muscle. After the internal opening of the fistula has been identified, a small strip of mucous membrane and lining of the anal canal is excised, giving contact to the

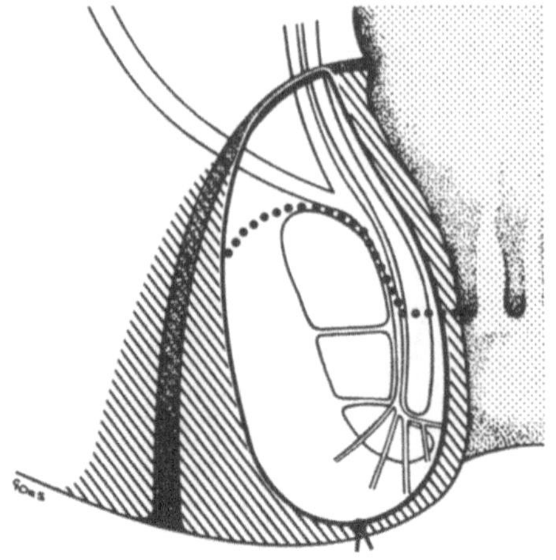

Fig. 6. An extrasphincteric fistula is treated by excision of the intralevatoric portion of the tract, the mucous membrane and skin layer from the inner opening to the external wound (*hatched area*). A seton is knotted tightly avoiding any traction

wound outside. The circular rectal muscle layer and internal sphincter is visible but not damaged. A nonabsorbable monofilament nylon thread is inserted through the short remaining fistula. It is knotted tightly so that the thread lies on the muscle, but does not cause tension. Follow-up visits regularly take place every 2 weeks in the outpatient clinic. When the seton is no longer visible on rectoscopy, i.e. the mucosa has grown over the thread and the inner opening is closed, the seton can be removed.

Results

In the last 10 years, we treated 199 patients with fistula-in-ano [25]. Eighteen were suffering from Crohn's disease and 26 demonstrated a complex fistula-in-ano as defined at the beginning of this paper. In one of these 26 the diagnosis of Crohn's disease was subsequently established. Incontinence developed only in one patient.

Fourteen of the 26 patients with complex fistulas were treated with a seton (Table 1). After an average of 6 weeks, the seton was removed in all cases. The patient with a complex fistula and Crohn's disease presented with an extrasphincteric fistula and was treated by the above-mentioned method. The fistula healed with no recurrence in the past 6 years, but a diverting colostomy had to be established because of a severe proctitis. In one patient, drainage of a horseshoe abscess resulted in a suprasphincteric fistula with one internal and three external openings. Treatment by the seton method was successful, but there slight faecal discharge remained.

In eight patients with a high trans-sphincteric fistula, three of these fistulas healed without any complications. Five experienced recurrences 2–3 months after removal of the seton. In two, a new seton was placed successfully, and two were treated by laying open the fistula, resulting in one with

Table 1. Results of treatment using a seton in 14 patients with a complex fistula-in-ano

Type of fistula	*n*	Primarily healed	Recurrence	Second type of treatment	Healed	Faecal discharge	Lost to follow-up
extrasphincteric	1	1	–	–	–	–	–
suprasphincteric	1	1	–	–	–	1[a]	–
trans-sphincteric							
high	8	3	5			–	
				seton	2 } 4	–	–
				fistulotomy	2	1	1
				refused	1	1	
low	4	1				–	
			3	fistulotomy	3	1	2
Total	14	6	8		8	4	3

[a] Three external openings

persistent faecal discharge. One was lost to follow-up, and one who was still suffering from slight discharge refused a further operation.

In the remaining four patients a trans-sphincteric fistula running from the dentate line was treated by a seton, because simple fistulotomy was judged too risky in a rather short anal canal. In one patient, it healed without complications while in three recurrences developed again 2–3 months after removal of the seton. They all were reoperated on by fistulotomy: in one a second intersphincteric fistula was laid open during the same operation, resulting in persistent slight faecal discharge, in the other two, the fistulas healed, but the patients lost to follow-up.

Discussion

Treatment of complex fistula-in-ano remains a challenge for the surgeon. Many different operations have been proposed, some of which are presented and discussed in this book. Our results are limited to the use of a seton with the aim of encouraging the internal opening to close using the two-stage operation proposed by Parks and Stitz [21].

We are not aware of any publication that proposes the use of a seton in the same way as we do. This method does no damage to the sphincter muscles in cases where healing cannot be achieved. However, in six of 14 patients, healing was obtained at the first attempt and there was no complication, except in one with a suprasphincteric fistula resulting from a horseshoe abscess with three external openings (Table 1). It is unclear if in this case discharge is due to the seton procedure rather than the treatment of the three external holes. Two more threads were placed in a second attempt, followed by an uneventful course. It is unsure if prolonged insertion of the seton would reduce the recurrence rate. However, recurrences always occurred after a 2- to 3-month interval and not immediately after removal. A healing time of 6 weeks is not unusual. Seventy-seven per cent of our 199 wounds after operation for fistula-in-ano were closed within 2 months [25].

All our patients treated with fistulotomy as a second procedure and with follow-up are still suffering from continuous but slight faecal discharge, sometimes causing a perianal dermatitis. The deformity of the anal canal seems to be significant, and reconstruction of the sphincter may need to be considered in patients with perianal skin problems, although they would be continent for semisolid stool and flatus.

Our method of using a seton as a drain to allow the closure of the internal fistula opening is worthwhile in fistulas that run from above the dentate line, although in some cases two attempts had to be made. However, the aim of producing fibrous tissue is valid even in a short anal canal to avoid a lot of persistent discharge or even incontinence. Therefore we recommend our technique of putting a seton in patients with complex fistula-in-ano as a successful method of treatment, and in some patients when a further operation may be required.

Discussion

Akovbiantz: Can you cut just the lower part of the external sphincter in trans-sphincteric fistulae?

Thomson: Perhaps I did not state my practice clearly enough. The patients that we were reporting on were those where the primary track was at the level of the line of anal valves or above, not below. Where the primary track crosses below the line of the anal valves, then I am sure it is quite safe to cut the lower part of the external sphincter.

Hardcastle: Could Dr Buchmann give us a few more details about the management of a seton? How long does he keep it in?

Buchmann: We leave it in for an average of 6 weeks. We have had eight failures in 14 patients, and the recurrences have occurred after 2–3 months. We remove the seton when we believe the track has closed around the seton completely.

Marti: The seton probably ought to be of fine material such as 40 or 50, otherwise it can be uncomfortable for the patient. Once healing has occurred around the seton, we close the internal opening with a sliding advancement flap.

Buchmann: I think the sliding advancement flap is a good technique, but not to be done in the acute phase.

Marti: No, after 2 weeks.

Mortensen: May I enquire about the effect of division of the internal sphincter on function. The internal sphincter is a very important structure for the maintenance of continence. We know that after dorsal sphincterotomy there may be incontinence.

Thomson: I think the incontinence caused by dorsal sphincterotomy which results from the guttering is in fact soiling rather than true incontinence. We recently looked at a series of patients with lateral sphincterotomy where 10% of the patients complained of soiling (unpublished data). I feel confident that soiling is due to guttering even in lateral sphincterotomy patients. I think the reason why the resting pressure is probably not interfered with in fistula patients is that where there has been sepsis; if the fibrous tissue is not excised, it holds the internal sphincter more or less together, and does not, therefore, spring apart as it would do in uninflamed tissue. This is the only explanation I can offer.

Marti: The most important part of the internal sphincter is the upper part, so the resting tone should not be greatly changed if only the lower part is divided. When treating fissures, I never take my sphincterotomy higher than the line of the anal valves.

Buchmann: Minor degrees of incontinence can be treated by anal sphincter repair without a covering colostomy and might be appropriate in these patients.

Lane: I agree with what has been said by the panel that we are moving towards a more conservative approach in fistula surgery. I am a little worried in my own mind that in adopting the core-out procedure I might be missing side tracks. If anal ultrasound or fistulography were routinely used, perhaps this would not happen. I wonder what views the panel have if they did not have access to these new investigations.

Marti: I do not think that you would leave any tracks behind if you follow the basic principles even if you do not have the sophisticated investigations.

Is There a Place for a Diverting Colostomy in Patients with Complex Fistula?

Buchmann: I think that a colostomy is only needed to overcome severe inflammation in the pelvis and around the anus, especially in patients with Crohn's disease.

Marti: I think we should distinguish between cellulitis of the pelvis and a fistula track.

Buchmann: I do not think a colostomy is required for nearly all fistulas, only for an associated very large abscess with cellulitis.

Akovbiantz: We never use a colostomy, but I think it may be required in some patients with extrasphincteric and suprasphincteric fistula. Arnold in Wiesbaden (Germany) cuts out the fistula in an extrasphincteric fashion, constructs a colostomy and then does a type of York-Mason repair on the sphincters. He has done this in 62 patients, but I have not seen his results published yet.

Hardcastle: I find that one needs to use a colostomy very rarely indeed. Perhaps in traumatic cases and in those with extrasphincteric tracks it is appropriate.

References

1. Law PJ, Talbot RW, Bartram CI, Northover JMA (1989) Anal endosonography in the evaluation of perianal sepsis and fistula in ano. Br J Surg 76: 752–755
2. Seow C, Burnett S, Bartram CI, Nicholls RJ (1990) A comparison between ultrasound digital examination in perianal fistulae. Gut 31: A604
3. Buchan R, Grace RH (1973) Anorectal suppuration: the results of treatment and the factors influencing the recurrence rate. Br J Surg 60: 537–540
4. Wilson DH (1964) The late results of anorectal abscess treated by incision, curettage and primary suture under antibiotic cover. Br J Surg 51: 823–831
5. Ellis M (1960) Incision and primary suture of abscesses of the anal region. Proc R Soc Med 53: 652–653
6. Page RE, Freeman R (1977) Superficial sepsis: the antibiotic of choice for blind treatment. Br J Surg 64: 181–184
7. Nesselrod JP (1949) Anal canal and rectum. In: Christopher F (ed) A textbook of surgery, 5th edn. Saunders, Philadelphia, p. 1092
8. Eisenhammer S (1956) The internal anal sphincter and the anorectal abscess. Surg Gynecol Obstet 103: 501–506
9. Eisenhammer S (1958) A new approach to the anorectal fistulous abscess based on the high intermuscular lesion. Surg Gynecol Obstet 106: 595–599
10. Eisenhammer S (1961) The anorectal and anovulval fistulous abscess. Surg Gynecol Obstet 113: 519–520
11. Parks AG (1961) Pathogenesis and treatment of fistula-in-ano. Br Med J 1: 463–469
12. Wilson GS, Miles A (1975) Principles of bacteriology, virology and immunity, 6th edn. Edward Arnold, London, p. 2607
13. Grace RH, Harper IA, Thompson RG (1982) Anorectal sepsis: microbiology in relation to fistula-in-ano. Br J Surg 69: 401–403
14. Whitehead SM, Leach RD, Eykyn SJ, Phillips I (1982) The aetiology of perirectal sepsis. Br J Surg 69: 166–168
15. Eykyn SJ, Grace RH (1986) The relevance of microbiology in the management of anorectal sepsis. Ann R Coll Surg Engl 68: 237–239

16. Henrichsen S, Christiansen J (1986) Incidence of fistula-in-ano complicating anorectal sepsis: a prospective study. Br J Surg 73: 371–372
17. Kronberg O (1985) To lay open or excise a fistula in ano, a randomized trial. Br J Surg 72: 970
18. Mann CV, Clifton MA (1985) Re-routing of the track for treatment of high anal and ano-rectal fistulae. Br J Surg 72: 134–137
19. Thomson JP, Ross AH (1989) Can the external anal sphincter be preserved in the treatment of trans-sphincteric fistula-in-ano? Int J Colorect Dis 4: 247–250
20. Parks AG, Gordon PH, Hardcastle JD (1976) A classification of fistula-in-ano. Br J Surg 63: 1–12
20a. Arnous J, Parnaud E, Denis J (1972) Quelques réflexions sur les abcès et les fistules à l'anus. Rev Prat 22: 1793–1814
21. Parks AG, Stitz RW (1976) The treatment of high fistula in ano. Dis Colon Rectum 19: 487–499
22. Marti MC (1990) Anorectal abscesses and fistulas. In: Marti MC, Givel JC (eds) Surgery of anorectal diseases. Springer Berlin Heidelberg New York
23. Buchmann P (1988) Lehrbuch der Proktologie, 2nd edn. Huber, Bern
24. Weber E, Buchmann P (1982) Eröffnung anorectaler Abscesse – mit oder ohne Fistelspaltung? Chirurg 53: 270–272
25. Hirth G (1990) Analfisteln. Therapie und Langzeitergebnisse. Thesis, University of Zurich

Part VII: Posters

Internal Anal Sphincter Electromyography: Correlation with Resting Anal Pressure

G.S. DUTHIE and D.C.C. BARTOLO

Little is known about the electromyographic (EMG) activity of the internal anal sphincter (IAS) in vivo, in man. IAS activity is responsible for approximately 80% of resting anal canal pressure (RP), but EMG activity is said to correlate poorly with RP. To determine the relationship of IAS activity and RP, we have recorded RP (air filled manometry system) synchronously with IAS EMG (frequency range 0.1–15 H_3) both at rest and during rectoanal inhibitory reflex testing (RAIR) in 26 patients (10 men, 15 women). RP (median, 62.5 cm H_2O; range, 15–150) failed to correlate with EMG amplitude (median, 0.22 mV; range, 0.10–0.45; $r = 0.156$; $p > 0.1$), but correlated with EMG frequency (median, 0.38 H_2; range, 0.21–0.62; $r = 0.829$; $p < 0.001$). To corroborate this relationship, the reduction in RP, EMG amplitude and EMG frequency were studied during RAIR. Decrease in RP (median, 40 cm H_2O; range, 10–90) failed to correlate with decreased EMG amplitude (median, 0.10 mV; range, 0–0.40; $r = 0.445$; $p > 0.05$), but correlated with decrease in EMG frequency (median, 0.24 H_2; range, 0.04–0.50; $r = 0.850$; $p < 0.001$). We conclude that the IAS component of RP is related to EMG activity, but this is frequency and not amplitude related.

Pelvic Floor Neuropathy in Diabetic Patients with Faecal Incontinence

M. Pinna Pintor, G.P. Zara, E. Falletto, L. Monge and M. Demattei

Anorectal sensory and motor function were compared in two groups of diabetic patients affected by peripheral somatic neuropathy, one group consisting of six patients with faecal incontinence (group A), the other of eight patients without faecal incontinence (group B) and in ten healthy control subjects (group C).

Anorectal manometry showed a slight increase in resting pressure in group B (67.8 ± 12 mmHg) compared with groups A (51.7 ± 23 mmHg) and C (53.2 ± 17 mmHg).

Pressure reached the normal range, with voluntary contraction, in groups B (129 ± 16 mmHg) and C (129 ± 22 mmHg), but not in group A (93 ± 33 mmHg). In group A, voluntary contraction could not be sustained for more than 4.6 ± 3 s, in comparison with longer period in groups B (16.3 ± 6 s) and C (17 ± 6 s).

Pudendal nerve terminal motor latencies, expressed as the mean of left and right sides, showed raised values in all the patients in group A (3.26 ± 1.3 ms) and in four patients in group B (2.39 ± 0.7 ms). The differences between these two groups and group C (1.94 ± 0.006 ms) were analysed by the Fisher exact test: A vs C, $p < 0.001$ and B vs C, $p < 0.0229$.

We conclude that faecal incontinence in diabetic patients might be related to somatic neuropathy of the pudendal nerve. Impairment of pudendal nerve terminal motor latencies is frequent in diabetics with peripheral neuropathy, but there is a need for prospective studies to define if this test is a predictive marker of diabetic incontinence.

Pouch Pressure Waves and Low Nocturnal Anal Pressure Are Related to Nocturnal Leakage After Restorative Proctocolectomy

G.S. DUTHIE and D.C.C. BARTOLO

Restorative proctocolectomy is occasionally associated with faecal leakage, especially at night. This has been seen in patients with high pressure pouch waves. We have investigated anal canal and pouch pressures by compressed, computerised ambulatory monitoring in ten controls (C), ten continent pouch patients (CON) and five with nocturnal leakage (INC) over prolonged periods (median 13.5 h; range 7–25) to determine changes in pressure profiles associated with leakage. Average daytime anal pressures were similar in all groups (for C, the median was 66 cm H_2O, the range 37–121; for CON, the median was 54.5 cm H_2O, the range 47–73; for INC, the median was 54.5 cm H_2O, the range 47–73) but controls had higher nocturnal pressures ($p < 0.01$; for C, median 24 cm H_2O, range 16–42; for CON, median 16 cm H_2O, range 6–28; for INC, median 10 cm H_2O, the range 0–62). Nocturnal pressure was significantly lower than daytime pressures in all groups ($p < 0.001$). High pouch pressure waves were seen in four incontinent and one continent patient. These were mirrored by anal pressure increases. Pouch pressure (median 113 cm H_2O, range 74–121) approximated anal pressure (median 114 cm H_2O, range 104–131) during the day, and was lower at night (median 89 cm H_2O, range, 40–138 vs median 97 cm H_2O, range 36–132). At night, pouch pressure exceeded anal pressure on 25% of occasions, but not in the daytime, nor in the continent patient with high pressure waves. Average pouch wave frequency was 5 per hour. In conclusion, there is a marked drop in anal pressure during sleep in all individuals. Pouch pressure waves are associated with leakage, but only at night does the pouch pressure ever exceed the anal pressure response.

Small-Bowel Transit Time Estimation Following Restorative Proctocolectomy

W.A. Kmiot, J.D. O'Brien and M.R.B. Keighley

Measurement of small-bowel transit time (SBTT) by breath hydrogen estimation is based on caecal anaerobic bacterial fermentation of luminal substrate. The high anaerobic counts in ileal reservoirs have led us to study the influence of SBTT on functional outcome in 12 patients (6 J pouches and 6 W pouches) at a median (95% CI) of 20 (range 12–33) months following restorative proctocolectomy.

All subjects ingested 30 ml lactulose in 400 ml chicken soup and 100 ml of dilute barium solution. The meal was followed radiographically and the time of the head of the meal appearance in the pouch compared with the first peak obtained by concurrent breath hydrogen testing (BH). Validation studies in normal subjects ($n = 10$) showed that BH and radiographic transit (RT) were highly correlated: RT, median (95% CI) 72, (46–96) min versus BH, median (95% CI) 70 (40–80) min; $r = 0.92$ (Spearman rank correlation); $p < 0.001$. However, BH and RT were not correlated in pouch patients: RT, median (95% CI) 28 (23–33) min versus BH, median (95% CI) 20 (0–30) min; $r = 0.284$ according to Spearman rank correlation. This was due to poor association of BH and RT in six subjects. Two had early BH peaks whilst the meal was in the jejunum. The remaining four failed to produce any hydrogen because of low counts of anaerobes: no BH median (95% CI) 2 × 10 (0–6 × 10) CFU/ml compared with median (95% CI) 6.5 × 10 (1 × 10–1.8 × 10) CFU/ml in patients producing hydrogen. A more rapid RT was associated with an increased 24-h defaecation frequency in pouches ($r = -0.79$; $p < 0.010$), but pouch design did not influence RT (J pouch median 26 (23–58) min versus W pouch median 29 (17–24) min; not significant according to the Wilcoxon two-sample test.

These data demonstrate that decreased SBTT after restorative proctocolectomy may contribute to high defaecation frequency, but that BH estimation is unreliable due to the variability of pouch anaerobic bacterial counts.

The Aetiology of Acute Reservoir Ileitis (Pouchitis): Is It Due to Faecal Stasis?

W.A. KMIOT and M.R.B. KEIGHLEY

Pouchitis may be due to faecal stasis or as a result of impaired pouch emptying and high anal sphincter pressures. We have studied pouch emptying and anal manometry in the aetiology of pouchitis.

Anal manometry, saline infusion test and evacuation pouchography were performed in 30 patients: pouchitis (P; $n = 10$), no pouchitis with poor function (NPP; $n = 10$), and no pouchitis with good function (NPG; $n = 10$). Maximum resting anal pressure was no different between P [median (95% Cl) 103 (85–130) cm H_2O] and NPG [median (95% Cl) 105 (90–130) cm H_2O], but both were significantly higher than NPP [median (95% Cl) 88 (80–100) cm H_2O] $p = 0.017$ using one-way rank analysis of variance]. Maximum squeeze anal pressure was not significantly different between the three groups [P, median (95% Cl) 140 (115–190) cm H_2O, NPP, median (95% Cl) 142 (90–180) cm H_2O; and NPG, median (95% Cl) 145 (120–220) cm H_2O; $p = 0.71$]. No patient had an intact rectoanal inhibitory reflex. Pouch volume at first leak of saline was also not significantly different between the groups [P, median (95% Cl) 150 (120–440) ml; NPP, median (95% Cl) 305 (100–1000) ml; NPG, median (95% Cl) 365 (200–1000) ml; $p = 0.24$ using one way rank analysis of variance]. Pouch emptying was not significantly different between the three groups (P, median 72 (4–92)%; NPB, median 43 (8–75)%; NPG, median 87% (0–100)%; $p = 0.24$ using one-way rank analysis of variance) and the ano-pouch angle widened to a similar extent during defaecation throughout all groups [P, median (95% Cl) 133°, (110°–155°); NPB, median (95% Cl) 128 (115°–140°); NPG, median (95% Cl) 123°, (105°–140°); $p = 0.76$].

This study does not provide any evidence to support the hypothesis that either impaired pouch emptying or increased anal sphincter pressures are associated with the aetiology of pouchitis.

Colostomy Is a Safe Procedure in a District General Hospital

M.C. Parker, J. Jamieson, S. Morris and C.G. Marks

There is controversy between ileostomy and colostomy for faecal diversion. In our hospital colostomy (loop or end) has been the method of choice and we present the results in 139 patients between 1980 and 1985.

There were 51 elective and 88 emergency procedures with mean ages of 65.3 years (range 38–84) for elective and 69.7 years (range 40–92) for emergencies. Seventy-three operations were for cancer, 40 emergencies; 46 were for diverticular disease, 37 emergencies; 20 operations were performed for other reasons. Twenty-six per cent of patients undergoing elective formation of colostomy had complications, but only six had stoma problems requiring revision. Thirty-four of 88 emergencies (39%) had complications, but only two of ten with stoma problems required surgery. There were ten deaths (7%), seven emergencies and three in the elective group, but none related to stomal problems. Following closure of colostomy (87 patients) there were four transient faecal fistulas but no deaths.

Colostomy is a safe procedure in a district general hospital with 6% of patients requiring revision surgery and with a low mortality due to co-existing disease.

Hartmann's Procedure: A Worthwhile Option?

A.R. Dixon and J. Thornton Holmes

Between January 1983 and January 1988, 32 patients (age range 40–91 years, median 67 years) with colorectal carcinoma underwent a Hartmann procedure. Twenty operations were performed as emergencies, the indications being obstruction or peritonitis, and 12 were elective operations. Of 22 surviving patients with potentially curable resections, 17 had a stapled restoration of colorectal continuity without complication. Five patients refused this option. Of the nine palliative procedures, seven patients developed a pelvic recurrence, one metastatic disease and the remaining patient died of an unrelated illness.

The median hospital stay was 17 days (range 8–48). There were two post-operative deaths (6%), both from pulmonary emboli. Thrombotic events occurred in a further three patients and wound sepsis in four. Other complications inherent to this procedure were individual cases of pelvic sepsis, anastomotic stricture and failed initial attempt at reversal.

These findings confirm that this operation is safe and effective in dealing with rectal and distal sigmoid colon malignancies with potential for local recurrence and in patients presenting as an emergency with obstruction or peritonitis.

Vaginal Fistulae Following Ileoanal Pouch Surgery: A Troublesome Complication

T.C.B. DEHN, M.J.McC. MORTENSEN and M.G.W. KETTLEWELL

Pouch-vaginal fistula (PVF) is an uncommon, but unpleasant, complication following ileoanal pouch construction. It is not only difficult to manage but may necessitate pouch excision. We report here on three cases of PVF in a consecutive series of 76 pouches (4%) and one referred case. The median age of the patients was 22 (19–44) years.

Three patients had undergone peranal mucosal proctectomy and all had peranally sutured pouch-anal anastomoses and loop ileostomies. Vaginal discharge commenced within 2 weeks postoperatively in three patients and at 7 months in one patient. Partial anastomotic separation occurred in two patients. In all four patients the level of fistula was at the pouch-anal anastomosis – the level of vaginal opening being similar in three and at the vulva in one.

Table 1 indicates the operative procedures required to achieve resolution of the fistulae. The median time between pouch construction and resolution/pouch excision was 29 (11–38) months. Following our experience, we suggest early repair by vaginal advancement flap followed, if necessary, by fistulotomy and subsequent sphincter repair. Stapled anastomosis without mucosal proctectomy may prevent fistulae arising secondary to peranal suturing difficulties.

Table 1. Operative procedures to resolve fistulae

Patient	Operative procedure	Outcome
1	Simple suture; fistulotomy; sphincter repair	Pouch excision (inadequate sphincter)
2	Simple suture; vaginal advancement flap ×4	Successful
3	Vaginal advancement flap ×3 fistulotomy; sphincter repair	Successful
4	Defunctioned; pouch reconstruction	Pouch excision (Crohn's disease)

In Vivo Measurement of Human Colorectal Tumour, Adenoma and Normal Mucosa Proliferation Using Flow Cytometry and Bromodeoxyuridine

D.A. Rew, I. Taylor, P.C. Weaver and G.D. Wilson

Until recently, the need to use radioisotopes has handicapped efforts to understand the in vivo cell kinetics of human tumours. Flow cytometric analysis of human tissues which have been pulse-labelled with the drug 5-bromo-2-deoxyuridine (BRdU) has been reported. Simultaneous measurements of nuclear BRdU content and total nuclear DNA content on a flow cytometer yield a measure of the DNA ploidy, the total and aneuploid labelling indices (LI), the duration of the S phase of the tissue cell cycle (Ts) and the potential doubling time of the tumour (Tpot).

An intravenous injection of 250 mg BRdU was given to 97 patients with colorectal adenocarcinomas 2.4–6 h prior to surgery. There were 49 colonic and 51 rectal tumours. Three patients had synchronous tumours. Multiple specimen blocks were studied from 61 of the 100 tumours. Fifty-two of 100 tumours were aneuploid (ploidy range 1.1–2.4). The mean total LI was 9.0% (range 0.6–22.2%) and the mean aneuploid LI was 12.2% (range 1.0–25.5%). The Ts and Tpot were calculated in 98 tumours. The range of the Ts was 4.0–28.6 h, with a mean value of 14.1 h. The mean Tpot was 5.9 days (range 1.7–21.4 days).

The crypt LI and crypt turnover rate (CTR) were estimated from flow cytometric data in 147 normal mucosal specimens of ileum, colon and rectum at least 10 cm from the primary tumour. All were diploid, with a mean crypt LI of 2.9% (range 0.8–15.2%). The mean CTR was 14.7 days (range 1.7–55.8 days). There was no change in mucosal proliferation detected along the tract. Four villous adenomas were studied. All were diploid. The mean LI was 5.0% (range 2.3–9.1%).

There was no correlation between the tumour LI Ts or Tpot and the degree of tumour differentiation or the Dukes stage. It is too early to assess the relationship of these data to clinical outcome.

The measurement of tumour and tissue proliferation can now be performed safely and reproducibly in vivo. This method may lead to new prognostic indicators and therapies based on a better understanding of colorectal mucosa and tumour cell proliferation.

Is Local Excision Appropriate for Early Rectal Carcinoma?

P. CASSELL

Conservation of the anal sphincter whilst accomplishing adequate resection of rectal cancer has become the surgical objective over the past few years. Most recent studies show that more patients have an anterior resection than abdomino-perineal excision of the rectum.

A further conservative trend has involved the management of the small group of patients with early invasive cancer in the lowest 10 cm of the rectum. Peranal excision of the cancer has been associated with low morbidity and good survival. Most of the patients so treated have been elderly, but many studies have reported a few younger patients.

Our experience with the elderly has been favourable, but the outcome in the two patients under 55 years of age we studied was uniformly bad. In each a complete excision of an early invasive cancer with well-differentiated histology had been carried out. In one patient, posterior rectal lymphadenopathy became apparent after 3 years despite no local recurrence. Excision of the rectum, however, did not prevent death from metastases within a few months. The second patient had local recurrence after 2.5 years. Again despite rectal excision, boney metastases developed within 18 months.

We question whether the younger patient should be treated by local excision because in a minority either there could at the time be lymphatic spread or ultimately local recurrence which even the delayed radical excision may not cure.

Dukes A patients overall have an excellent prognosis. The highly selected group suitable for a "curative" local excision should be at the best end of the spectrum (although a minority will ultimately prove to be Dukes C). For the younger patient the morbidity of rectal excision is, we believe, preferable to the risk of not offering the patient the best chance of cure.

A Comparison of an Immunological and a Chemical Faecal Occult Blood Test in Symptomatic Patients

J.D. Hardcastle, W.M. Thomas and G. Pye

Immunological tests for faecal occult blood may show enhanced sensitivity for colorectal neoplasia. We have compared the immunological test Hemeselect (Smith-Kline, USA) with the well-established chemical test Haemoccult (Rohm Pharma) in consecutive patients with lower gastro-intestinal symptoms.

Patients completed both tests prior to outpatient assessment; they subsequently underwent either colonoscopy or barium enema examination. Two hundred and sixty (96%) of 271 patients approached returned completed tests. Overall 12% of patients had at least one positive Haemoccult test and 28% a positive Hemeselect result. Thirty-five carcinomas were diagnosed, 21 (60%) were Haemoccult positive and 33 (94%) Hemeselect positive ($\chi^2 = 11.67, p < 0.01$). The increased sensitivity was particularly evident for the 11 cancers which were rectal, 5 (45%) being detected by Haemoccult and 11 (100%) by Hemeselect ($\chi^2 = 8.25, p < 0.01$). Three (37.5%) of eight patients with adenomas >1 cm in size were Haemoccult positive compared with five (62.5%) which were Hemeselect positive.

Hemeselect may have a role in identifying a group worthy of urgent investigation. Population-based studies are required to assess whether the enhanced sensitivity is maintained without an appreciable loss in specificity when used for colorectal cancer screening.

Beware of Haemolytic Uraemic Syndrome Presenting as Colorectal Disease in Adults

H. Thompson, A. Allan and M.R.B. Keighley

The haemolytic uraemic syndrome is seen occasionally by the surgeon in adult patients with colorectal manifestations [1, 2]. Our first case involved a 35-year-old housewife who presented as an emergency with clinical features resembling acute appendicitis. Laparotomy revealed that the appendix was normal, but the caecum was blue-black in colour. Right hemicolectomy was carried out, but the patient developed the clinical features of disseminated intravascular coagulation and renal failure during the postoperative period leading to death on the 15th day.

The second case involved a 51-year-old housewife who presented with abdominal pain and blood-stained diarrhoea. Stool cultures were negative, and sigmoidoscopy revealed a friable granular mucosa with contact bleeding indistinguishable from ulcerative colitis. Barium enema showed total colitis which was most severe in the descending and sigmoid colon. Dilatation of the colon developed on the third day and emergency colectomy was carried out. She deteriorated during the postoperative period with evidence of disseminated intravascular coagulation and renal failure. Death occurred 5 days after colectomy.

The diagnosis of the hemolytic uraemic syndrome was established at autopsy in the first case. Histological diagnosis of ischaemic colitis in the second case suggested that the underlying cause was the hemolytic uraemic syndrome.

References

1. Allan A, Keighley MRB, Thompson H (1989) Beware of hemolytic uremic syndrome presenting as colorectal disease in adults. Report of two cases. Dis Colon Rectum 32: 426–428
2. Anonymous (1987) Unravelling HUS (Annotation). Lancet ii: 1437–1439

Subject Index

GPSR Compliance

The European Union's (EU) General Product Safety Regulation (GPSR) is a set of rules that requires consumer products to be safe and our obligations to ensure this.

If you have any concerns about our products, you can contact us on ProductSafety@springernature.com

In case Publisher is established outside the EU, the EU authorized representative is:

Springer Nature Customer Service Center GmbH
Europaplatz 3
69115 Heidelberg, Germany

Batch number: 10704713

Printed by Printforce, the Netherlands